SUPERFOODS
for Babies and Children

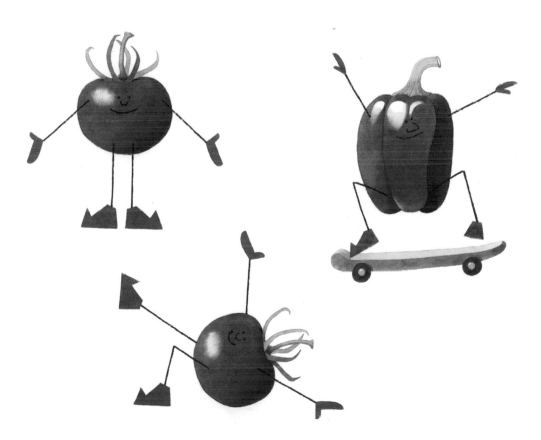

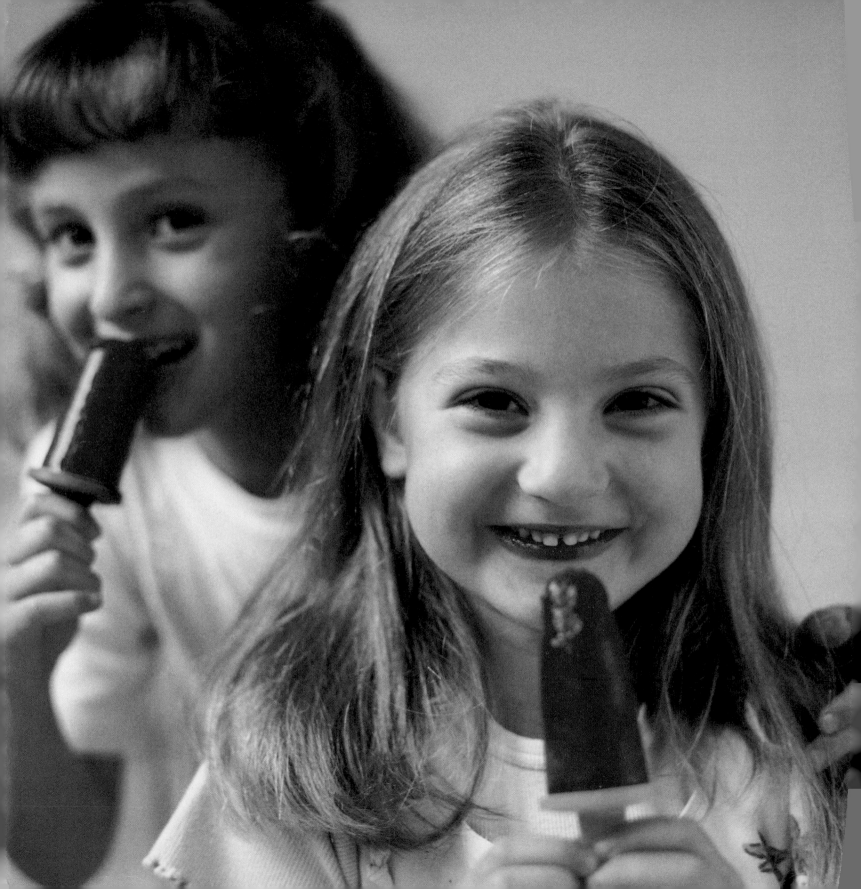

SUPERFOODS
for Babies and Children

Annabel Karmel

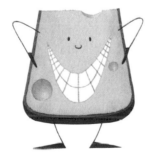

ATRIA PAPERBACK

New York London Toronto Sydney

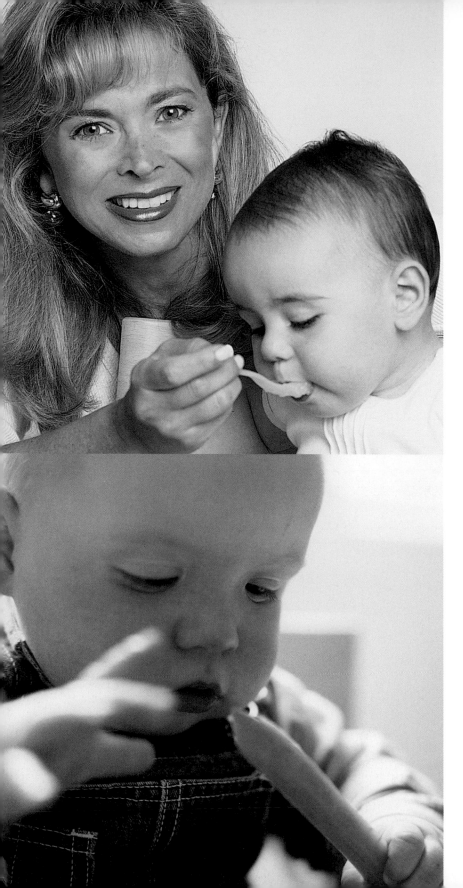

ATRIA PAPERBACK

A Division of Simon & Schuster, Inc.
1230 Avenue of the Americas
New York, NY 10020

Originally published in Great Britain in 2001 as
Annabel Karmel's SuperFoods for Babies and Children by Ebury Press

Published by arrangement with Cooking for Children Limited

First Atria Paperback edition January 2011

ATRIA PAPERBACK and colophon are trademarks of
Simon & Schuster, Inc.

For information about special discounts for bulk purchases,
please contact Simon & Schuster Special Sales at
1-866-506-1949 or business@simonandschuster.com.

The Simon & Schuster Speakers Bureau can bring authors
to your live event. For more information or to book an event,
contact the Simon & Schuster Speakers Bureau at
1-866-248-3049 or visit our website at www.simonspeakers.com.

Manufactured in the United States of America

10 9 8 7 6 5 4 3 2 1

The Library of Congress has cataloged the hardcover edition as follows:

Karmel, Annabel.
   Superfoods for babies and children / Annabel Karmel.
      p.   cm.
   1. Infants—Nutrition—Popular works.   2. Children—Nutrition—
Popular works.   3. Cookery (Baby foods).   I. Title.
RJ216.K367 2006
641.5'6222—dc22   2006041166

ISBN 978-0-7432-7522-4
ISBN 978-0-7432-7524-8 (pbk)
ISBN 978-1-4391-8385-4 (ebook)

contents

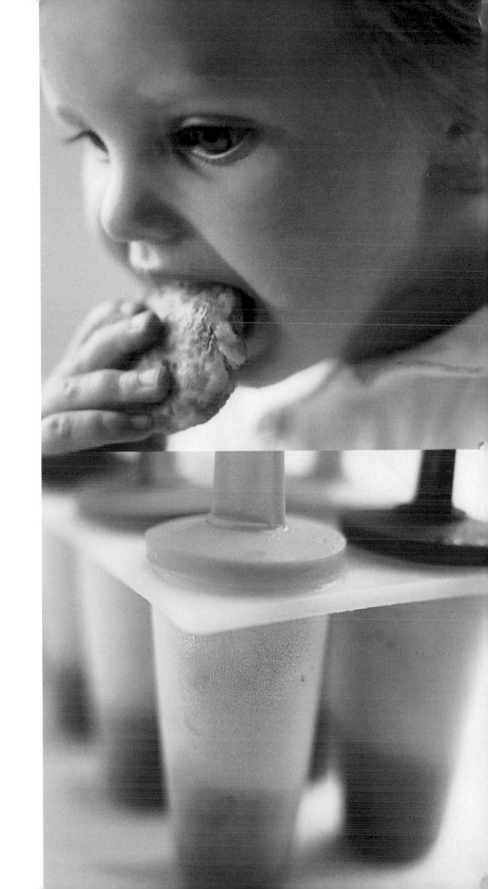

introduction

Feeding children can be one of the most frustrating aspects of child rearing. As parents we all start off with the best of intentions, but all too soon we find that our two-year-old wants only Thomas the Tank Engine pasta shapes or dinosaur chicken nuggets, and our six-year-old eats only Coco Pops. Frazzled to the core, we are all tempted to give in to the seductive television/magazine advertising where the perfect baby/child is seen remorselessly gobbling the last mouthful of a proprietary brand. It's shocking that at a time when diet is most crucial to health, the label "children's food" represents some of the worst-quality, most unhealthy food you can buy.

Many children go through a stage when all they seem to do is eat just a few foods or simply pick at their meal and push away the plate. The problem often seems to be that the more we coax our children into eating, the more stubborn they become and the less they eat. Toddler power comes of age!

American children are in the middle of a health crisis, and food is a contributing factor. Childhood obesity is on the rise, as is diabetes. So many of us will die from diet-related diseases, but by setting up a good diet in the vital first few years, you will help protect your child's future. Studies are now beginning to show that chronic diseases such as heart disease take root early in life. Having lost my first child, Natasha, due to a rare viral infection when she was very young, I became determined that my three children would grow up to enjoy eating good healthy food, since what they stuffed into their mouths was within my orbit of control and I felt I could make a difference.

Following Natasha's death, I wanted to channel my grief into something positive, but it wasn't until a year later that it became clear to me what form that would take. My second child, Nicholas, was born in rather fraught circumstances, delivered by my husband on the staircase. He was—not unnaturally—the apple of his mother's eye, and maybe my predilection for purees came out of this! It is actually thanks to Nicholas that I have my career, as he was the most terrible eater. He would eat yogurt and fruit but refused almost everything else with a stubbornness that belied his tender years. Since he refused jars of baby food, I resolved to make up my own recipes to tempt him. Having always had a passion for cooking, I decided that I could easily produce foods that tasted delicious and were much better for him than the processed purees you can buy in the supermarket.

Working with Great Ormond Street Hospital, where Natasha died, I produced my first book: *The Complete Baby and Toddler Meal Planner,* now an international best seller, which is designed to put the joy back into feeding children. All the recipes were tested on babies and toddlers to see exactly what it was that they enjoyed eating—after all, healthy food is all very well, but if children don't like it, then it's a wasted effort. Nicholas is now seventeen years old, and he and his sisters, Lara (sixteen) and Scarlett (thirteen), like to cook, and they eat nearly everything. They certainly keep me well in check with the views of the younger generation when it comes to culinary matters.

The power of fresh food

Why bother with making baby food? What's wrong with baby food from a jar, anyway? Take one of these jars and look carefully at the expiration date. The substance inside has been designed to last for two years past the date of purchase. To create a shelf-stable product, commercial baby food is heated to extremely high temperatures and then cooled, eliminating a lot of the nutrients and much of the flavor. Many brands also add thickeners and stabilizers. There is nothing wrong with giving babies prepared foods for the sake of convenience, but don't believe these preparations are a healthier option.

Children are much less likely to become fussy eaters if they are used to a good selection of fresh foods from an early age. With the children that I see, the picky eaters tend to be the ones brought up on jars of bland commercial purees, and the babies given fresh foods from the beginning easily make the transition to joining in with family meals.

The phenomenon of a separate diet for children—chicken nuggets, burgers, pizza—is relatively new. Many parents end up preparing separate meals for their child because he or she is so fussy. There was once a time—believe it or not—when children ate the same food as their parents. My aim has always been to find recipes that are quick and easy to prepare, and here is a collection of delicious, healthy recipes that can be enjoyed by the whole family.

Using the recipes

In addition to the SuperFoods information that stands alongside each recipe, the following symbols are used when they are relevant:

 a recipe you can freeze

 suitable for vegetarians

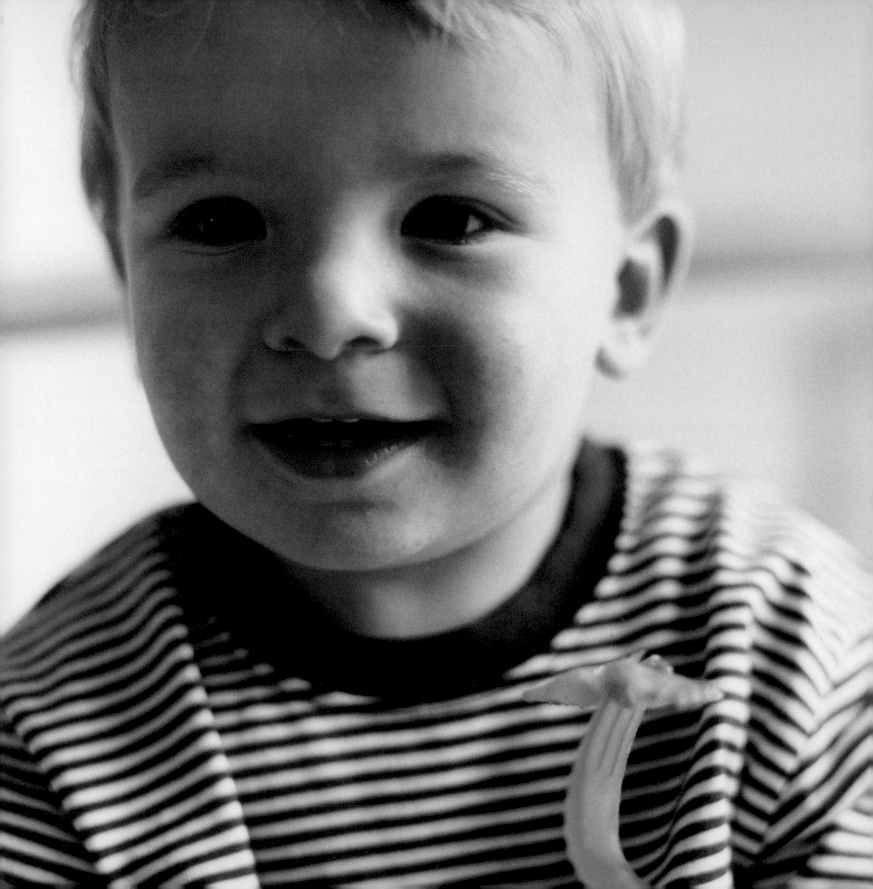

SuperFoods

What we feed our children today will determine their future tomorrow. A well-stocked pantry is the best form of preventive medicine known to man.

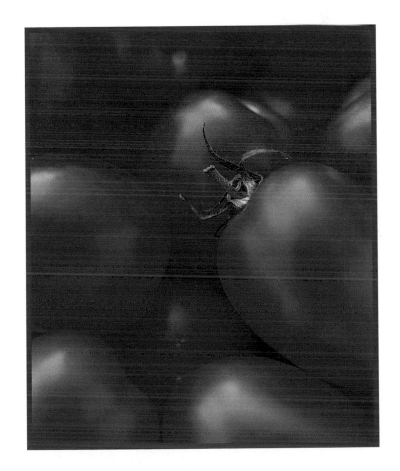

Eating by color

SuperFoods are foods that have roles other than supplying the basic components of our diet—carbohydrates, protein, and fat. These roles vary from boosting energy and brain power to prevention of illness and even repair of damage. Research shows that one-third of cancer cases are related to what we eat, and the evidence is that fiber and fresh fruit and vegetables are in surprisingly short supply in the Western diet. Researchers estimate that diets filled with fruits and vegetables instead of fats, along with exercise, could reduce cancer incidence by 30 to 40 percent.

So what exactly is it that makes SuperFoods so great? The answer is the chemical structures we know as vitamins, minerals, and trace elements, also known collectively as phytonutrients, one of nature's many miracles. Many fruits and vegetables are packed full of these powerful natural chemicals, which have very important functions in healing and preventing illness and diseases, such as cancer and heart disease.

The incidence of cancer is increasing tremendously in Western society, as well as the incidence of obesity among children. Fruit and vegetable consumption among schoolchildren is woefully low. The latest research shows that one in five young people aged four to eighteen eats no fruit or vegetables, and less than half have the recommended five portions a day. Eating at least five portions of fruit and vegetables per day is vital to good health, and we should be incorporating fruit and vegetables into our children's diet from a very young age so these foods become a completely normal part of life.

Another reason for the health-giving benefits of fruit and vegetables is the presence of antioxidants. These are a group of substances that include vitamins C and E; beta-carotene (the orange color found in plants), which the body converts into vitamin A; and the minerals iron, selenium, zinc, and copper. Antioxidants play a key role in protecting our bodies from the damage that can cause serious illness, particularly heart disease and cancer. Antioxidants effectively disarm certain harmful molecules known as free radicals, which can cause damage and disease. Many fruits and vegetables are rich in antioxidants, and the key to making sure you are getting a good supply of antioxidants is to choose a good variety of brightly colored fruits and vegetables to eat each day. The time to start stocking up with these protective nutrients is in childhood—it can never be too early.

The color of food

GREEN	RED	ORANGE/YELLOW	DARK BLUE/PURPLE	WHITE
asparagus	baked beans	apricots	beets	apples
avocados	cherries	cantaloupes	blackberries	cauliflower
broccoli	grapes	carrots	black currants	mushrooms
brussels sprouts	guava	lemons	blueberries	onions
cabbage	papaya	mangoes	eggplant	potatoes
fava beans	plums	oranges	grapes	
kale	raspberries	passion fruit	plums	
lettuce	red bell pepper	peaches	prunes	
peas	red/pink grapefruit	pumpkins		
spinach	strawberries	rutabagas		
watercress	tomatoes	squash		
	watermelon	sweet potatoes		

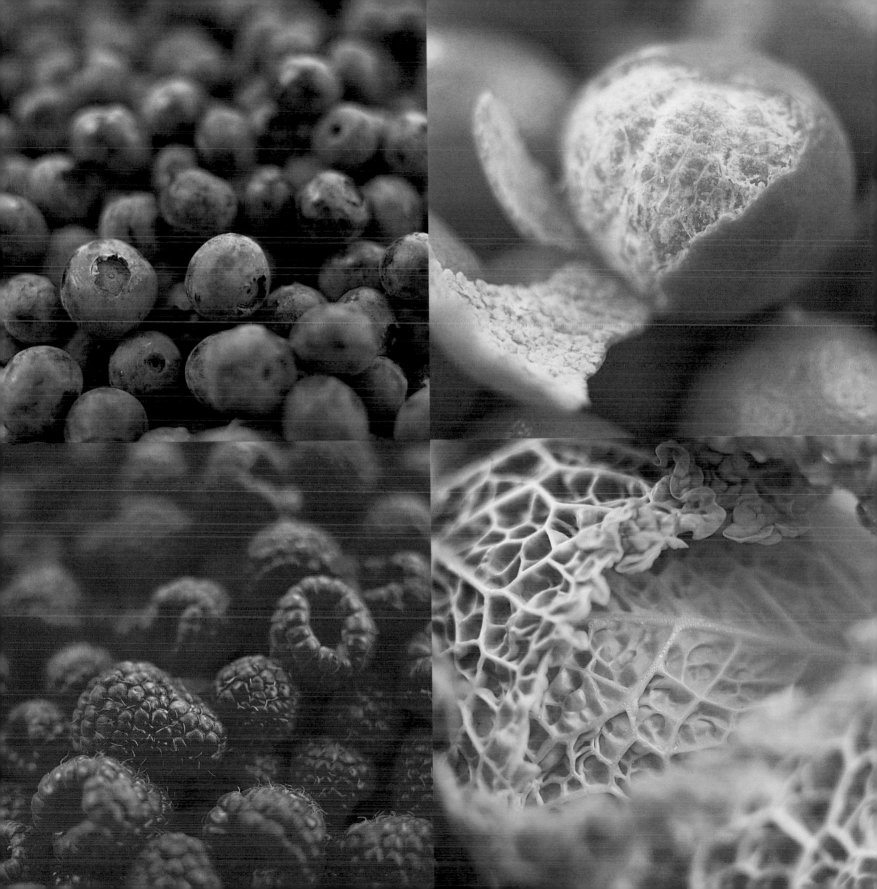

SuperFoods by color

It is easy to make sure children get all the SuperFoods they need, simply by using the lists of fruit and vegetables given on the previous page to plan colorful meals. Fire-engine red, sunshine yellow, emerald green, rich purples—these bright fruit and vegetable colors are not just feasts for our eyes, but treasure troves of healthy nutrients. For locked inside tomatoes, spinach, oranges, and blueberries are whole sets of plant nutrients that can reduce our risk of heart disease and cancer. In general, the more colorful the food, the more nutritious it is. For example, spinach rates more highly than lettuce, the deep orange of a sweet potato contains more nutrients than an ordinary potato, and pink grapefruit is preferable to an ordinary grapefruit. It is important to ensure that you include a good variety of colors to make sure you are getting a good balance in your diet.

Healthy eating: *For years nutritionists have emphasized the benefits of fresh fruit and vegetables. However, lycopene is easier for our bodies to absorb when the tomatoes have been processed or cooked with a little oil in foods like tomato soup and tomato sauce for pasta, and—good news—even ketchup is a good source.*

Green

Green foods are rich in the antioxidant vitamins A, C, and E, which can protect our bodies' cells and boost our chances of living a longer, healthier life. Green leafy vegetables are also rich in iron. The green color comes from chlorophyll, which is a plant's way of converting sunlight to energy. Studies have shown that regularly eating broccoli reduces the risk of cancer. It is also a good source of glucosinolates, which have strong anticancer effects by stimulating our bodies' natural defenses.

Red

Lycopene is a natural pigment that gives fruits like tomatoes, red grapefruits, and watermelons their red color and is one of the most powerful cancer-fighting carotenoids. It is particularly valuable in helping to protect us from certain cancers such as prostate and cervical cancer. Carotenoids are also found in carrots, dark green vegetables, red bell peppers, sweet potatoes, peaches and apricots (fresh and dried), mangoes, cantaloupes, and papayas.

Studies have revealed that men who had high levels of lycopene in their fat stores were half as likely to have a heart attack. Most of the lycopene in the diet comes from tomatoes because of the quantity of tomatoes and tomato products we eat. However, other good sources are watermelon, guava, and pink grapefruit. Lycopene is not produced by the body and needs to be derived from our diet.

Orange and yellow

Orange and yellow fruits and vegetables are high in beta-carotene, the plant form of vitamin A. It is true that vitamin A improves night vision, and during the Second World War it was rumored that fighter pilots were fed a diet of carrots so they could see better in the dark. Beta-carotene also protects against cancer and boosts the immune system against colds and flu. Citrus fruits are good sources of vitamin C, which is important for growth, healthy skin, healing wounds, and improving the absorption of iron.

Dark blue or purple

There is a lot of vitamin C as well as antioxidants such as bioflavonoids and ellagic acid in blue and purple foods, which help to boost immunities against cancer. Grapes in particular contain ellagic acid. The skins of grapes also contain a substance that can lower cholesterol and prevent fats in the bloodstream from sticking together. As a result, a daily glass of red wine is now thought to help lower cholesterol levels.

Beets are especially rich in iron and magnesium. The pigment anthocyanin (from the Greek for "dark blue flower") has powerful anticancer properties. Blueberries have one of the highest antioxidant levels of any fruit because of the high level of anthocyanin in the skin.

White

Just because you can't see it doesn't mean it isn't there. Garlic, onions, and leeks contain organosulphides, which seem to stimulate the immune system and fight cancer. Organosulphides are also antioxidants. Garlic is rich in allicin, which is an antibiotic and is antiviral.

Eating a balanced diet

To grow properly and keep healthy, children need to eat a good balanced diet. The food guide pyramid on page 15 has been designed to show the food groups that make up a balanced diet, and children should aim to achieve this balance by the age of five. Children under five need a diet higher in fat and lower in fiber because of their high energy requirements.

Carbohydrates

This group should make up the largest part of your child's diet. Bread, cereal, rice, and pasta are the body's main source of energy and also provide vitamins, minerals, and fiber. Whole-grain cereals and breads are also a good source of iron. Children should eat about five servings from this group each day.

....

Did you know? *Potatoes should not be counted as a vegetable portion. In fact, nutritionally they are classed as a starchy food along with bread and cereals, so your child should be eating five portions of fruit and vegetables a day on top of potatoes.*

Healthy eating: *Vitamin supplements contain only a small proportion of the nutritional benefits available from fruit and vegetables.*

Examples of what counts as one serving of carbohydrates

- One slice of bread.
- A small portion of rice or pasta.
- A small bowl of cereal.

Try to choose natural rather than refined carbohydrates (see page 19), such as brown rice, whole-wheat bread, legumes, and fruit. These foods release sugar relatively slowly into the bloodstream, which helps provide long-lasting energy. Unrefined carbohydrates are also a good source of vitamins, minerals, and fiber. Refined carbohydrates like white bread and white rice have lost many of their valuable nutrients during their processing. These foods still provide a good source of energy, but try also to include a good proportion of natural, unrefined carbohydrates in your child's diet.

Vegetables and fruits

Vegetables and fruits are important, as they provide phytochemicals such as vitamins and minerals, which help protect us against cancer and heart disease (see "Eating by color," page 10). Fruit and vegetables are also an important source of fiber. Different fruits and vegetables contain different vitamins, so it is important to include as much variety as possible. Vegetables, particularly root vegetables, also provide carbohydrates for energy. For the recommended five portions a day (see page 10), a three-year-old might have a tangerine, mandarin orange, or clementine, half an apple, four dried apricots, a tablespoon of peas, and a tomato throughout the day.

Dairy

These foods provide protein, vitamins, and minerals and are the best source of calcium, which is important for good health and the formation of bones and teeth. In the first year, milk forms a very important part of your child's diet. Between the ages of one and five, children should have approximately 20 ounces of milk a day or the equivalent in other dairy products. Children should have three portions of milk or dairy products each day. This could be a glass of milk, a serving of yogurt, or 1½ ounces of cheese (a matchbox-size piece).

Protein

Meat, poultry, fish, legumes, eggs, and nuts supply a good source of protein, which is important for the growth, maintenance, and repair of body tissue (see also "Growth foods," page 16). An inadequate supply of protein can lower resistance to infection. Meat, poultry, and fish also supply B vitamins, iron, and zinc.

Once your baby is eating three meals a day, try to make sure that she has some protein at two of these meals. Protein doesn't always have to be meat or fish; dairy products or a legume served with a cereal are a good source. An example would be rice and beans. As a rough guide, children should eat meat or chicken three to four times a week and two or more portions of fish a week, one of which should be an oily variety like tuna, sardines, or salmon. Protein foods like cheese or eggs are good for breakfast.

Fats and sugary processed foods

Children need proportionately more fat in their diet than adults, so for the first two years serve whole milk, cheese, and yogurt. Up to the age of one, children should derive 50 percent of their energy from fat (breast milk contains 50 percent fat). It provides a concentrated source of energy; fatty acids are important for brain and visual development (see page 17), and fats contain the fat-soluble vitamins A, D, E, and K.

You should try to ensure there is enough fat in your child's diet, but you should also seek to introduce healthy eating by choosing lean meat and cutting down on fried food. Milk and cheese are good sources of fat and they are also rich in calcium, protein, and vitamins. For adults and children over five, fat should provide no more than 30 percent of their calorie intake—cut down on junk food and processed foods like potato chips and cookies.

Vitamins and minerals

We are foolish if we think we can beat nature at its own game. Vitamin and mineral supplements can never hope to replace all the nutrients contained in food. Listed below are the main vitamins and minerals that children need to grow and be healthy.

Vitamins

Vitamins are essential for the maintenance of a healthy body. Vitamins are either water-soluble (vitamins B and C) or fat-soluble (A, D, E, and K). Water-soluble vitamins, except for vitamin B_{12}, cannot be stored in the body, so foods containing these should be eaten regularly. These vitamins are destroyed by heat and dissolve in water, so do not overcook foods that contain them. Fat-soluble vitamins can be stored in the body, and excessive amounts accumulate and can be toxic. If a balanced diet is eaten, it is highly unlikely that this would happen, but beware of supplements.

Vitamin A: Also known as retinol, vitamin A only occurs in animal foods, but fruit and vegetables contain carotenoids, which are converted to vitamin A by our bodies. Important for growth, preventing infections of the nose, throat, and lungs, healthy skin, and good night vision, vitamin A is found in liver, oily fish, whole milk and cheese, butter, margarine, and egg yolks.

B complex vitamins: These are important for growth and the development of a healthy nervous system and are essential for converting food into energy. No foods except liver and brewer's yeast extract contain all of the vitamins in the B group. Good

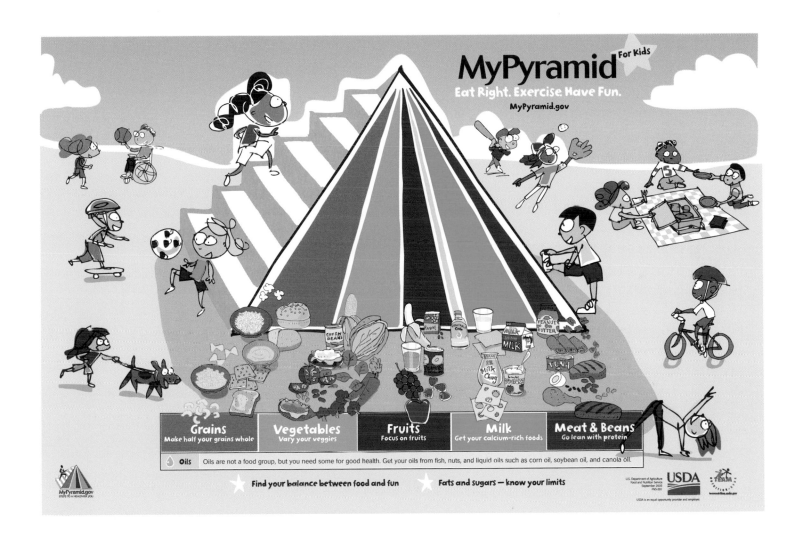

sources are meat, dairy products, eggs, sardines, dark green leafy vegetables, whole-grain cereals, tofu, and nuts.

Vitamin C: This vitamin cannot be produced by our bodies and is needed for the growth and repair of body tissues, healthy skin, and the healing of wounds. It is also important because it helps the body absorb iron and is a powerful antioxidant. Good sources are citrus fruits, strawberries, kiwifruit, black currants, bell peppers, broccoli, dark green leafy vegetables, and chile peppers.

Vitamin D: Although this is found in a few foods it is mainly manufactured by the skin when it is exposed to sunlight. This is one of the reasons why children should try to get some fresh air every day. It is needed to absorb calcium and phosphorus for healthy bones and teeth and to avoid rickets. Good sources are oily fish such as tuna, salmon, and sardines, milk and dairy products, eggs, and margarine.

Vitamin E: This is needed to help develop and maintain strong cells, protect against heart disease, and maintain good function in the nervous system, and it may be important in maintaining immunity. Good sources of vitamin E are vegetable oil, wheat germ, avocado, nuts, and seeds.

Vitamin supplements: *Give a vitamin supplement of A, C, and D from the age of 6 months if your baby is being breast-fed or is drinking less than 18 ounces of infant formula a day. Ask your pediatrician for advice.*

Minerals

There are many minerals in food and of these, iron and zinc are very important. Selenium and copper are also essential to a well-rounded diet: They are both antioxidants, which means they help prevent damage to cells from free radicals (see page 10). Good sources of selenium include whole grains, nuts, meat, poultry, and fish. Good sources of copper are whole-grain cereals, bread and pasta, and dried fruit, tofu, legumes, nuts, and seeds.

Iron: Iron deficiency is the commonest nutritional deficiency in the Western world. Babies are born with a store of iron that lasts for about the first six months. When this store of iron is depleted, a baby must obtain sufficient iron from the diet. There are a few types of iron, the best source of which is found in meat and is easily absorbed by the body. Plant food sources are more difficult to absorb and the third type, added by manufacturers to foods such as breakfast cereals, is absorbed less well. However, if foods or drinks containing vitamin C are eaten at the same meal, then the iron is better absorbed. Offer fresh fruits like kiwis, citrus, or berry fruits for dessert or a small glass of pure fruit juice. A good combination for breakfast would be an iron-fortified cereal followed by kiwifruit and strawberries.

Zinc: In general, dark red meat has a higher zinc content than white meat, and fish has less than meat. Cereals are a good source of zinc, but as it is contained in the outer layer of the grain, the more refined the cereal, the less zinc there is. Good sources include red meat, whole-wheat bread, Cheddar cheese, lentils, shellfish, pumpkinseeds, and fortified breakfast cereals.

Growth foods

Children grow and develop rapidly. Protein is the building block of all the cells in our bodies and therefore an essential part of the diet. Since children grow so quickly, they have a higher requirement for protein than do adults. As well as helping growth, proteins are also important for repairing any damage to body tissue. It is reassuring to know that protein deficiency is almost unheard of in the United States, and most of us eat more protein than we need.

Protein is made up of amino acids, some of which the body can manufacture and some of which can be obtained from food. Animal proteins contain all the amino acids that the body needs, whereas soy is the only plant-based food that contains all the essential amino acids. To obtain complete proteins, legumes and grains need to be combined, such as peanut butter on toast or lentils and rice. Good animal sources of protein are red meat, poultry, fish, eggs, milk, cheese, grains, legumes, and tofu.

Fats and oils

Fats and oils are also included in this group of growth foods, not for their essential fatty acid properties but for their high caloric contents. Fats are like liquid gold packed full of energy. In order to meet the high demands for energy of a growing infant or child, the diet must contain adequate amounts of fat.

Babies and young children need more fat in their diet than adults because of their rapid growth, so don't be worried about adding a good dollop of butter to a baked potato or making pasta in a creamy cheese sauce.

Brain foods

Eggs are rich in choline, a B vitamin that is a key component in the brain transmitter acetylcholine, which is crucial for memory. There are many important factors in brain development but no scientifically proven links with specific types of food. That said, a balanced and varied diet and a good breakfast obviously ensures that all possible factors important for brain development are

....

Did you know? *Research suggests that a diet rich in omega-6 and omega-3 acids may improve the performance of children with attention deficit disorder, hyperactivity, or dyspraxia.*

present, and there are some foods that are better than others for stimulating the brain cells.

Natural starches

Although weighing only 2 percent of total body weight, the brain uses approximately 20 percent of the body's energy at rest. The brain's energy stores are very small, so to keep it functioning at its best it needs fuel, sugar, which is derived from carbohydrates. When levels of sugar in the blood fluctuate, behavior and learning become erratic. The best foods to keep blood sugars steady for the brain are the complex carbohydrates that contain natural starches (see page 19) and so supply a steady source of fuel, such as oatmeal, whole-grain cereal, brown rice, and sweet potatoes.

Iron

Foods that contain iron have been shown to prevent anemia, a condition that leads to tiredness, decreased mental alertness, lowered IQ, and overall apathy. Iron is also important for transporting oxygen in hemoglobin in our red blood cells to all organs in the body, including our brain; therefore iron is vital for good brain function. High-iron foods are red meat, liver, dried fruit, and iron-enriched cereals, such as shredded wheat.

Fatty acids

In the first year of life, a baby's brain grows at a very fast rate, generally tripling in size by the first birthday. Fats are a major component of the brain—this is one of the reasons why 50 percent of the calories of breast milk are composed of fat.

Oily fish like salmon, mackerel, tuna, and sardines are good brain boosters. This is due to their high levels of omega-3 essential fats, which optimize messaging between nerve cells in the brain. Good intakes are crucial for normal brain functioning in children and can sometimes improve problems like dyslexia and hyperactivity. There are two essential types of fatty acids that have been shown to be important for brain and visual development. They are alpha-linolenic (omega-3) and linoleic (omega-6) acids.

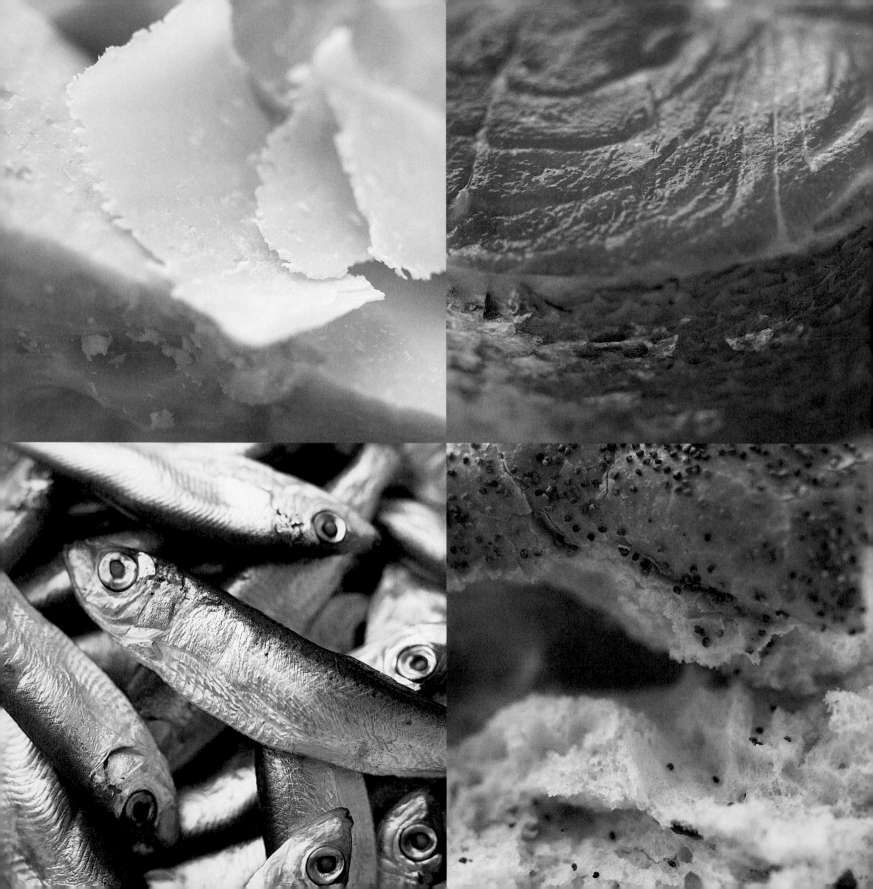

Foods rich in omega-3 are linseed oil, walnut oil, salmon, tuna, trout, and sardines. Foods rich in omega-6 are safflower oil, grapeseed oil, sunflower oil, and soft polyunsaturated margarine. Some foods are fortified with omega-3 oils, like certain spreads and some breads.

Energy-boosting foods

Foods containing carbohydrates are the main providers of energy in the diet. There are two types of carbohydrates: sugars (simple carbohydrates) and starches (complex carbohydrates), each of which can be found in two forms: natural and refined.

- Natural sugars are found in fruits and fruit juices.
- Refined sugars, including white and brown sugar and honey, are found in cakes, cookies, and soft drinks.
- Natural starches are found in whole-grain breakfast cereals, whole-wheat flour and bread, brown rice, potatoes, rolled oats, lentils, bananas, and root vegetables.
- Refined starches are found in white flour and white bread, sugary processed breakfast cereals, white rice, white pasta, cookies, and cakes.

All carbohydrates taken in by the body have to be digested and converted into glucose—a type of sugar. Of these, the natural carbohydrates provide the best source of energy, as they keep blood sugar levels constant because they release their sugar content into the bloodstream slowly, thus giving long-lasting energy. They also retain their vitamins, minerals, and fiber, so try to include some whole grain versions like brown rice and whole-wheat bread in the diet.

Healthy eating: *It is best to wash fruit but leave the skin on fruits like apples or peaches, as a lot of the nutrients lie just below the skin.*

Healthy eating: *If your child needs energy for a soccer match or sports event, it is best to give a meal based on foods that release sugar slowly into the bloodstream such as brown rice, pasta, whole-grain cereals, vegetables, and fruit. A good snack might be peanut butter sandwiches on whole-wheat bread or a banana. Give water or pure fruit juice instead of soft drinks. The sugar in soft drinks could trigger low blood sugar, leaving your child feeling tired. After physical activity and particularly in hot weather don't let your child wait until he feels thirsty to give him a drink. The chances are that he will already be dehydrated.*

Starchy foods like potato, rice, pasta, and bread provide energy at a slower rate than sugary foods. Refined sugars are quickly absorbed by the body, so energy levels rise dramatically for a short while. However, the problem is that the pancreas then produces lots of insulin in a bid to break down the sugar, which can lead to a rapid decline in energy. Fruit sugars provide quick energy but do not cause such a rapid rise and fall in energy because the fiber slows the absorption of the sugars.

The consumption of high-sugar foods and drinks like cookies, cakes, and soft drinks causes a rapid rise in blood sugar that can result in the body overcompensating, which leads to a dip in blood sugar levels, resulting in low levels of physical and mental energy. Instead, for sustained energy it is much better to choose fresh fruit, nuts and seeds, rice cakes, or nutritious sandwiches made with whole-wheat bread. With these foods in your diet, your energy levels will remain far more consistent and your concentration on a more even keel.

A good vegetarian diet

More and more families with children are choosing to become vegetarian, and a balanced vegetarian diet can be very healthy. However, it is important not to give up meat without replacing the nutrients that meat provides, particularly protein, iron, zinc, and possibly some B vitamins.

Adults' and children's diets do not always follow the same guidelines and whereas a fairly bulky high-fiber vegetarian diet might suit adults, it is not suitable for young children who are growing, as it can replace more energy-dense foods such as fat and carbohydrates. Also a lot of fiber in the diet can inhibit the absorption of minerals such as zinc, iron, and calcium and is very bulky and filling and can even cause toddler diarrhea.

Bringing up a baby on a vegetarian diet with a good volume of either breast milk or infant formula can provide all the nutrients she needs.

The importance of protein

Protein supplies your child with amino acids, essential chemicals that are the body's building blocks. While all animal proteins, including eggs and dairy products, provide a high-quality protein containing all the essential amino acids, cereals and vegetable proteins (such as peas, beans, lentils, and nuts and seeds) have a lower quality. Soy is the only plant-based food that contains all the amino acids.

To ensure your child gets a high-quality protein at each meal try to combine a cereal food, such as pasta, bread, or rice, together with eggs, dairy products like cheese, legumes, or nuts. Good ideas are peanut butter on toast, lentil soup with a whole-wheat roll, peanut butter sandwiches, baked potato with cheese and milk, and pasta with cheese sauce. Good vegetarian sources of protein include eggs, milk, cheese, yogurt, soy, beans, lentils, nuts, and seeds.

Examples of good protein combinations

- A cereal food such as pasta, bread, or rice with eggs, cheese, legumes, or nuts.
- Peanut butter on toast.
- Baked potato with cheese and milk.
- Pasta with cheese sauce.

The importance of iron

It is important to make sure that children brought up on a vegetarian diet have an adequate supply of iron (see page 16). Good vegetarian sources of iron include fortified breakfast cereals, egg yolk, whole-wheat bread, beans and lentils, dark green leafy vegetables, and dried fruit, especially apricots and peaches. Iron is absorbed more efficiently by the body if combined with vitamin C, so offer a food or drink high in vitamin C at each meal.

The importance of calcium

Calcium is important for the health and formation of bones and teeth, and breast or formula milk contains all the calcium that your baby needs. However, from six months you can introduce cow's milk and dairy products as a food (see pages 28, 68, and 92). Other good vegetarian sources of calcium are tofu (calcium fortified), dried figs and apricots, nuts, sesame seeds and hummus, and fortified soy milk.

B vitamins

Vitamin B_{12} is needed for growth and division of cells. It is only found in foods of animal origin such as meat, poultry, fish, eggs, and dairy produce. Some breakfast cereals are also fortified with vitamin B_{12}. Vegetarians can obtain sufficient vitamin B_{12} from eggs and dairy products.

Vegan diet

If you plan to follow a vegan diet, you should plan your child's diet carefully, in consultation with a pediatric dietitian (contact the American Dietetic Association for more information).

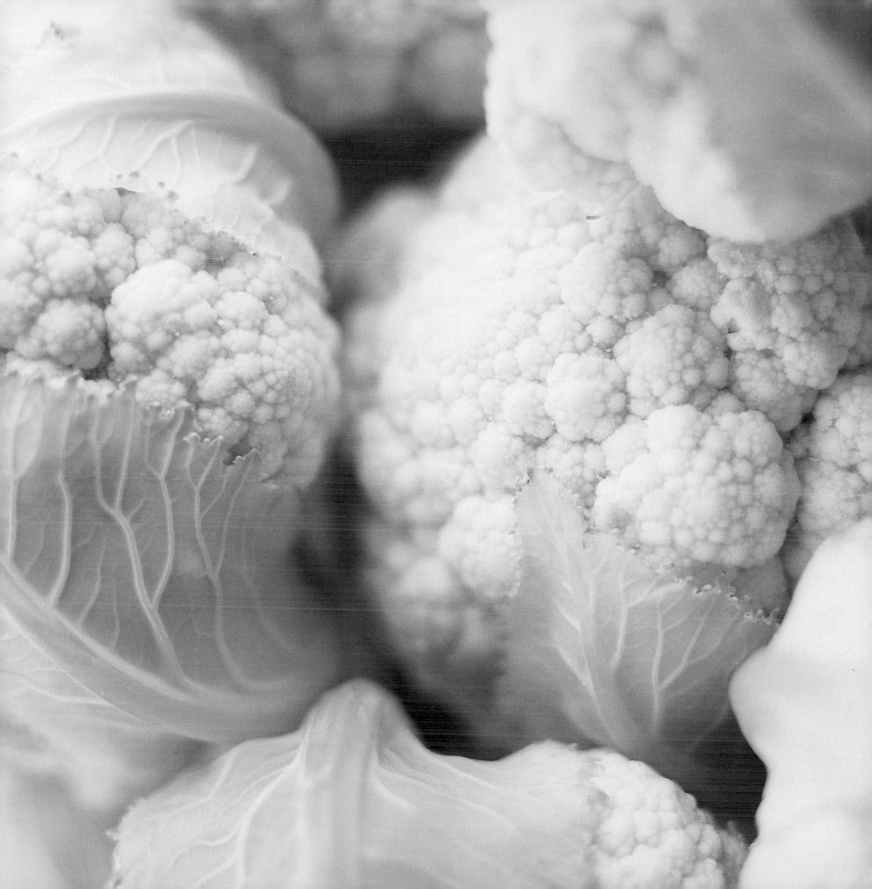

Shopping for food

Food labels list ingredients in order of decreasing weight. Try to choose foods that are low in sugar, salt, and saturated fat and avoid large amounts of colorings and artificial flavorings.

What is a little and what is a lot:

per 100 g of food	high	low
SUGAR	10 g	2 g
FAT	20 g	3 g
SATURATED FAT	5 g	1 g
FIBER	3 g	0.5 g
SODIUM	0.5 g	0.1 g

Fat and fiber

The amount of fat and fiber is not really an issue, as very young children need a more nutrient-dense diet with more fat and less fiber. However, from two years upward, children should gradually move toward an adult-type diet. When looking at labels, it is useful to check that the amount of saturated fat is not a large percentage of the total fat. There are two main types of fat: saturated fat derived mainly from animal sources, such as butter, lard, and the fat in meat and dairy products; and unsaturated fat, such as vegetable oil. As a general rule vegetable fats are healthier than animal fats, with the exception of fish oils in fish like salmon and sardines.

Salt

Too much salt in the diet may contribute to high blood pressure, which can increase the risk of a stroke, coronary heart disease, and kidney disease. It is therefore a good idea for the whole family to become accustomed to less salt in the diet. Try not to add too much salt while cooking and avoid salt on the table.

Babies under one year should not have any salt added to their food, as a baby's kidneys are too immature to cope with added salt. Toddlers (age one to three) should have no more than 2 g of salt (about ⅓ teaspoon) per day and a four- to six-year-old should have no more than 3 g of salt a day. Three-quarters of the salt we eat comes from processed foods like pasta, sausages and burgers, pizza, SpaghettiOs, and potato chips.

Sugar

Labels often break carbohydrates into starch and sugars, and it is useful to know that 5 g sugar makes 1 teaspoon. However, in many cases, because of poor labeling, it is impossible to establish the sugar content of sweet foods. Beware: Many foods marketed for children, such as breakfast cereals and cereal bars, may contain more than 35 percent sugar.

Sugar may come in many disguises, such as sucrose, glucose, glucose syrup, maltose, dextrose, fructose, corn syrup, high fructose corn syrup, honey, and fruit juices. And manufacturers can hide the amount of sugar in a product by using three different types of sugar, such as sugar, corn syrup, and honey, and by listing each sugar separately. Each appears lower down the list, making it more difficult to judge the total amount of sugar in the product. The term "no added sugar" can also be misleading, for the product could still contain honey, glucose, corn syrup, and concentrated apple juice, which are just as harmful as sugar to your child's teeth.

Most soft drinks are packed with sugar. A can of Coke or similar fizzy drink can contain 1¼–1½ ounces sugar, which is equivalent to about 8 teaspoons. Take care when choosing fruit juices, as pure unsweetened juices should contain no added sugars except the ½ ounce per liter that manufacturers are allowed. There are some individual cartons of fruit juice on the market that contain 1 ounce sugar, which represents more than 6 teaspoons sugar, and even fruit sugars will cause tooth decay. Likewise, watch out for juice drinks, which can contain as little as 5 percent juice.

Yogurts are a good source of calcium, but despite their healthy image, many yogurts contain a lot of added sugar, thickeners, colors, and flavorings. Similarly, many breakfast cereals designed to appeal to children can contain as much as 50 percent sugar. It would be much better for your child to start the day with a good old-fashioned cereal like oatmeal or muesli, even if your child adds honey or a little sugar.

Foods and drinks for babies and young children are not allowed to contain artificial sweeteners. However, these are included in many foods specifically targeted at youngsters—such as soft drinks, yogurts, and ice pops—disguised by technical jargon. When doing the weekly shopping, look carefully at the ingredients of what you are buying and beware if they include acesulfame k, aspartame, saccharin, or sorbitol, which are, in fact, artificial sweeteners.

Frozen food

In some cases, processed foods actually retain more nutrients than the unprocessed form. Perhaps the best example of this is frozen vegetables and fruits, which are picked and frozen within hours of harvest, thus locking in valuable nutrients. Fresh vegetables and fruits may have been stored for long periods before purchase or use, and the longer they remain on the shelf or in cold storage the more nutrients they lose. However, research has shown that frozen vegetables and fruits are just as good for you, if not better than their fresh relations.

Keep a good supply of frozen fruit and vegetables, such as peas, spinach, corn, summer berries, and thick-cut oven fries, in stock in your freezer. They make good standbys, they don't go moldy, and they are inexpensive and quick and easy to prepare.

Canned food

The process of canning preserves food by heating it to a sufficiently high temperature and replacing the oxygen with inactive gases and then sealing it in an airtight container to prevent microbial contamination. Most canned foods will keep almost indefinitely, and they retain many nutrients, including protein and vitamins A and D and riboflavin.

The high temperatures involved in canning tend to destroy vitamin B_1 and vitamin C in vegetables. But canned fruit and fruit juices tend to retain most of their vitamins. Most acidic foods retain their vitamin C content, so canned tomatoes are still good for you. Be aware that foods canned in brine are high in salt. Fruits canned

Healthy eating: *Manufacturers add vitamins and minerals to a variety of foods aimed at children, from sugary refined breakfast cereals to canned pasta and ice pops. It is a mistake to believe that adding vitamins to an otherwise unhealthy food will make it healthy, but sadly for a large percentage of children this source of vitamins, calcium, and iron is very important.*

in syrup are high in sugar, so instead choose fruits canned in natural juice.

Convenience food

Whereas many frozen meals are high in salt and fat, there are quite a number of convenience foods that are good to have on hand (see the suggestions on page 24).

Organic foods

Organic baby foods have grown in popularity as people have become increasingly concerned about the effects of pesticides and other agricultural chemicals on children's health. Organic farming is an environmentally friendly option, but it generates higher prices, and parents should not feel that a nonorganic diet is unhealthy. The risk of not including fruits and vegetables in children's diets is far greater, and there is no scientific evidence that pesticide levels in ordinary fruit and vegetables are harmful to babies and young children.

Organic food is grown in soil without the use of artificial fertilizers or pesticides and instead uses traditional crop rotation where possible and makes the most of natural fertilizers. Animals are reared without the routine use of antibiotics, growth hormones, or worming injections. The animals reared must also

Convenience foods worth stocking

- A good-quality ready-made tomato sauce.
- Fresh soup in cartons.
- Baked beans.
- Pizza with a vegetable and cheese topping.
- Good-quality ready-made pasta sauces.
- Pita bread and tuna to make a tuna salad pita pocket.
- Canned tuna, salmon, and sardines.
- Peanut butter.
- Dried fruits, such as apricots, figs, and prunes.
- Ready-made dips, such as hummus, guacamole, and sour cream.
- Cream cheese dips.
- Nuts and raisins.
- Good-quality ice cream.
- Frozen peas.
- Frozen leaf spinach.
- Frozen corn.
- Thick-cut frozen oven fries.
- Frozen berry fruits.

GM foods: Are these the new SuperFoods?

There is a great deal of controversy about the introduction of genetically modified (GM) crops and foods. Genetically engineering food is a new way of producing foods by taking DNA from one species and inserting it into another. One benefit of this would be that genetic modification could be used to enhance the protein content of rice—the lack of protein is a major cause of illness in many third world countries.

Unlike conventional breeding, where genes can only be transferred between plants or animals of the same or closely related species, genetic engineering enables genes to be transferred between different species and potentially even between animals and plants. For example, work is under way to produce plants with a built-in mechanism to fight frost damage. One possibility would involve utilizing the genes in fish that enable them to tolerate extreme cold.

It is virtually impossible to completely avoid GM foods in the United States. Many products containing soy, corn, or canola or any of their derivatives (fats and oils, etc.) come from GM crops, and there are almost no labeling requirements in the United States.

Many people are worried that the long-term effects of eating genetically modified food are as yet unknown and could be harmful to the environment.

be allowed to live natural, contented lives. However, pesticides have been used for so many years that they may still be present in the soil, water, and air. Spray drift of chemicals from neighboring farms make it impossible to guarantee that organic food is free from pesticide residues.

There is no law—and it is unlikely to occur—to say that organic produce must taste better. If you choose to go organic, you will need to shop at least two or three times a week, as there are no chemical preservatives in organic food, and fruit and vegetables in particular will deteriorate more quickly.

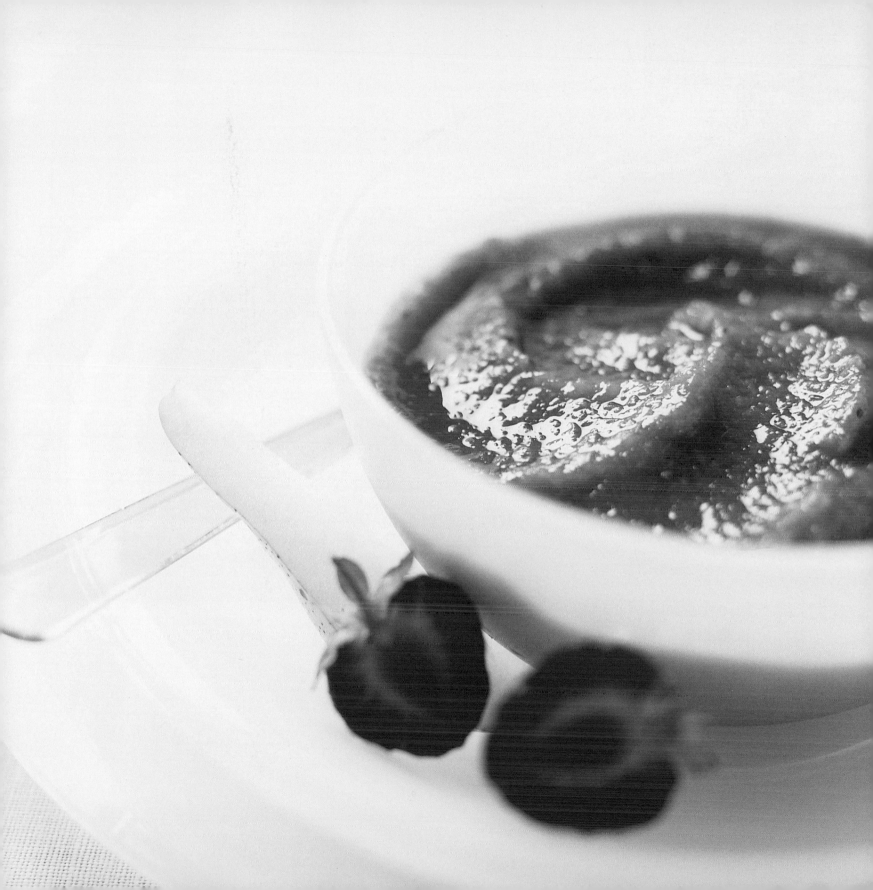

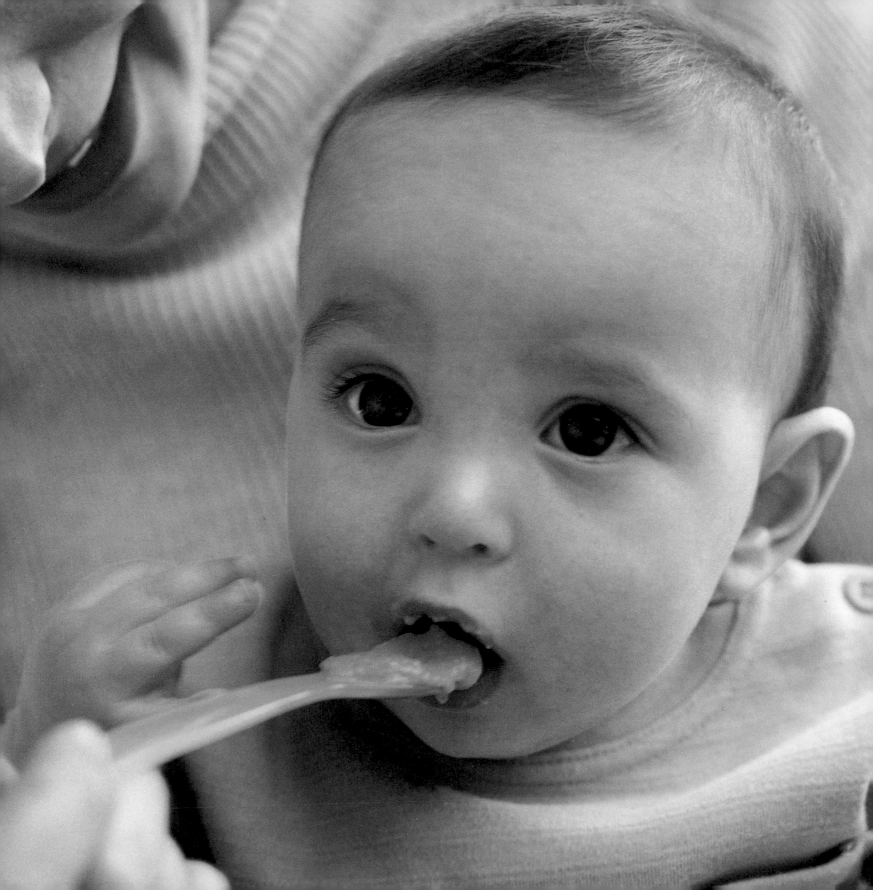

6 months:
the best first foods for your baby

Weaning your baby is an exciting time for both of you. It's a huge step forward for your baby into a whole new world of tastes and textures.

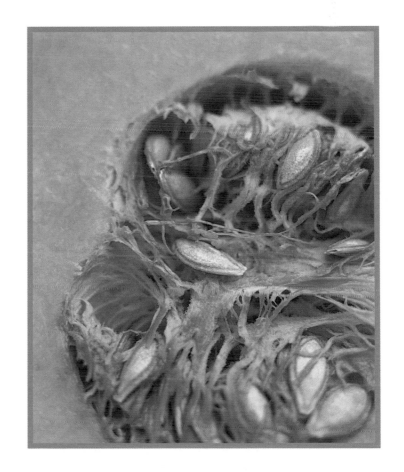

Breast-feeding benefits

For the first six months of life, babies need nothing more than milk, as this provides all the energy and nutrients that they need. Breast milk contains particular proteins called antibodies and white blood cells, which help to protect a baby from infection. Breast milk is also rich in the omega-3 essential fatty acids that are important for brain development. There is evidence that breast-feeding for thirteen weeks or more reduces the incidence of gastroenteritis and respiratory infections. Breast-feeding has been shown to delay the onset and reduce the severity of allergies in children from families with a history of asthma, hay fever, eczema, and food allergies. The colostrum that a mother produces in the first few days of breast-feeding is a very important source of antibodies, so there is a benefit in breast-feeding even for a short period. For a mother the benefits of breast-feeding include a lower risk of ovarian cancer and breast cancer. Furthermore, a baby's suckling at the breast causes the uterus to contract so that it returns to its normal size much faster.

Healthy eating: *Infant formula has amounts of nutrients, minerals, and vitamins similar to that of breast milk but none of the properties breast milk has to protect against infection. In breast milk, the amount of minerals available such as iron and zinc is excellent.*

How much milk?

Between four and six months, babies should have between 21 and 28 ounces of milk a day, and from the age of six months to one year, babies should have between 17 and 28 ounces of milk each day, mostly in the form of breast milk or formula milk. Although you can use cow's milk in cooking and with breakfast cereals, breast milk or formula should remain your baby's main drink, as these contain nutrients that cow's milk lacks, such as iron and vitamin C. Do not fill up your baby with solid foods at the expense of milk. Avoid baby drinks such as juices, as the only fluid your baby needs is milk. If the weather is very hot and you

Daily milk consumption

Approximate Age	Number of Daily Feedings
1 to 2 weeks	7 to 8
2 to 6 weeks	6 to 7
2 months	5 to 6
3 months	5
6 months	4

feel your baby needs extra fluid, offer cooled boiled water. There is extra fluid in the food your baby is eating because purees have a high water content.

What milk?

Cow's, goat's, sheep's, soy (noninfant, carton), rice, and oat milks are not suitable as your baby's main drink before one year, as they do not contain enough iron and other nutrients for proper growth. Whole cow's milk can be used in cooking or with cereal from six months but should not be given as your baby's main drink before the age of one year.

Young babies have high energy and nutrient requirements, so skimmed milk should not be introduced before five years because it is very low in energy. However, 2% milk can be given from the age of two if your child is eating and growing well.

Baby formula has higher levels of iron, vitamin D, protein, and sodium than infant formulas. It should be given only from six months of age and is not intended to replace breast milk or regular infant formulas, which are suitable up to twelve months of age. However, these milks are nutritionally more suitable than cow's milk and are generally recommended for children who are at risk of iron deficiency. They may be used until twenty-four months of age.

Other drinks for your baby

The only drink except for breast or formula milk that your baby should have in the first six months is water. Cooled boiled tap water is best. Bottled mineral water can contain high concentrations of mineral salts, which are unsuitable for young babies. High levels of nitrates, sulfates, and fluoride should be avoided. Carbonated (fizzy) water is also unsuitable for babies.

Specially manufactured fruit and herbal drinks for babies can sometimes contain quite large amounts of sugar, which can lead to tooth decay. If you want to give your baby fruit juice, it is much better to squeeze your own or choose one that contains only natural fruit sugars. Orange juice is a good source of vitamin C, which will help your child to absorb iron. All fruit juices should be diluted five parts water to one part juice, as even natural fruit sugars can cause tooth decay. Try to confine drinks other than water or milk to mealtimes; fruit or herbal drinks can take away a young baby's appetite for more valuable foods at mealtimes.

Introducing solids

Don't be in a hurry to wean your baby onto solids. For the first six months, breast milk or formula provides all the nutrients your baby needs. At around six months, however, your baby will reach a stage at which she needs solid foods as well as milk in her diet, and if weaning is delayed beyond this time, some babies can have difficulty learning to chew and swallow food.

Signs that your baby is ready for solids
• He is still hungry after a full milk feeding.
• He starts waking more during the night demanding to be fed.
• He demands feedings more often.

Babies grow more rapidly in their first year than at any other time in their life. A lot of parents continue to give only fruit and vegetable purees for too long. Babies need meat, chicken, and fish introduced into their diet soon after they are six months old. Iron deficiency is the most common nutritional deficiency in babies. Babies are born with an iron store that lasts for about six months, and baby's iron requirements are particularly high between the ages of six months and two years. This is a critical time for the growth of the brain, and a lack of iron in the diet can lead to impaired mental development.

In the first year of life, a baby's brain grows at a very fast rate, generally tripling in size by the first birthday. A large proportion of the human brain is composed of fatty acids that also play an important role in vision and the development of the retina. Oily fish like salmon are one of the richest sources of essential fatty acids and should be given toward the end of the first month of introducing solids.

The best first foods for your baby
The first foods that you give your baby must be easy to digest and unlikely to provoke an allergic reaction. Don't be tempted to add salt or sugar to your baby's food, however bland. Salt may harm your baby's kidneys and sugar will encourage a sweet tooth.

For the first few weeks it is not a good idea to give mixtures of foods other than baby rice mixed with a fruit or vegetable puree. Weaning is a good time to discover if there are any foods that your baby does not tolerate well, and when foods are mixed together it is hard to tell which of them is causing a problem.

First vegetables: Carrot, potato, rutabaga, parsnip, butternut squash, and sweet potato (see pages 36 to 39). Root vegetables like carrots and sweet potatoes tend to be the most popular with very young babies, as they are sweet and smooth once pureed. After first tastes, you can start to introduce other vegetables like zucchini, cauliflower, broccoli, and peas.

First fruits: Apple, pear, banana, papaya, and avocado (see pages 40 to 42).

Baby rice: Mixed with water or breast or formula milk, baby rice is easily digested and its milky taste makes an easy transition to solids. Choose one that is sugar free. Baby rice combines well with both fruit and vegetable purees.

Meat: Pureed chicken, turkey, or beef can be included in a baby's diet and are good sources of iron. It's a good idea to combine them with root vegetables, as this helps to produce a texture that is much smoother and easier to swallow.

Fish: Introduce soft white fish—flounder or cod is ideal.

Foods to avoid

• Salt: Babies under a year should not have any salt added to their food, as this can strain immature kidneys and cause dehydration. A preference for salt can become established at an early age and eating too much salt may lead to high blood pressure later in life. Also avoid smoked foods.

• Sugar: Unless food is really tart, don't add sugar. Adding sugar is habit forming and increases the risk of tooth decay.

• Foods containing gluten: Wheat, oats, barley, and rye should not be introduced before 6 months. When buying baby cereals and zwiebacks before 6 months make sure they are gluten free. Baby rice is the safest to try at first.

• Raw or lightly cooked eggs: Eggs should not be given before 6 months (due to the risk of salmonella infection) and should be cooked until the yolk and white are solid.

• Unpasteurized cheeses: Brie, Camembert, and Danish Blue should not be offered before 12 months due to the risk of listeria infection.

• Shellfish: Do not give until your baby is at least one year old, due to the risk of food poisoning and potential allergy.

• Nuts: Chopped and whole nuts are not recommended before the age of 5 due to the risk of choking. There is also a risk of allergic reaction to nuts.

• Honey: Do not give to your baby before one year. **It can very occasionally contain a type of bacteria that can result in a potentially serious illness called infant botulism.**

When to give feedings

Try to make feeding a special time to share with your baby rather than a chore, and pick a time of day when you are not rushed or liable to be distracted. If possible, try to feed your baby around the same time every day to establish some kind of routine. Babies are used to food coming in a nonstop steady stream and sometimes find the gaps between spoonfuls annoying. For some babies, it may be a good idea to begin by giving a little milk before their solids so that they are not frantically hungry, or they may become frustrated. For the first few days a baby will probably have only a tiny amount—maybe one or two spoonfuls. Start with one feeding a day, probably around lunchtime, and gradually increase to about three feedings a day (breakfast, lunch, and supper) by five or six months (see my meal planners on pages 33 to 35). Always test the temperature of the food before giving it to your baby. Sit your baby on your lap or in a baby chair and try to make it an enjoyable experience by smiling and talking to your baby as you feed her.

Food rejection

Avoid making a fuss if your baby won't eat, and try to stay relaxed. Try reintroducing food after a couple of days if at first solids are refused, or prepare a runnier puree so that it is easier for your baby to swallow. You could also try dipping a clean finger in the puree and allowing your baby to suck it off your finger, as some babies don't like the feel of a spoon in their mouths to begin with. If your baby takes only a very little food, try not to make mealtimes too drawn out in an attempt to get him to eat more. Babies usually know when they have had enough.

Making baby food

By making baby food yourself, you can be sure of using only the best-quality ingredients without the need for thickeners or additives. It also works out much cheaper to make baby food at home rather than buying commercial brands. Introducing a wide range of foods is important in establishing a varied and healthy diet, and you can make up your own combinations to suit your baby. You have the choice of organic fruit and vegetables if you like (see page 23).

Judging quantities

It is difficult to predict how much a baby will eat, since all babies' appetites and needs are different. As a very rough guide you will probably find that at the beginning your baby will take only one or two tablespoons of puree from a small, shallow weaning spoon, so allow about 2-tablespoon ice-cube portions (see box). As your baby develops, probably the best advice is to offer your baby 5–6 tablespoons of puree and keep going until her interest starts to wane. Provided your baby is gaining weight and has plenty of energy, you can rest assured that she is doing fine. If your baby has an insatiable appetite and you are worried that she is overweight, then seek professional advice.

Texture

To begin with, purees should be quite runny, resembling the consistency of a thick soup, and made up of only one or two ingredients. Your baby's purees should not be made up with tap water that has not been boiled but only with the water from the bottom of the steamer or the cooking liquid if boiling vegetables in a saucepan. You can thin purees by adding extra cooking liquid or milk and thicken purees by stirring in a little baby rice.

What temperature?

A baby's mouth is more sensitive to heat than ours and food should be given at room temperature or lukewarm. If reheating food in a microwave, heat until piping hot all the way through, allow to cool, then stir thoroughly to get rid of any hot spots and check the temperature before giving it to your baby.

Hygiene

Very young babies are particularly vulnerable to the effects of food poisoning, so you should take great care in the preparation and storage of your baby's food. Warm milk is the perfect breeding ground for bacteria, so scrupulously wash and sterilize bottles, nipples, and feeding cup spouts for the first year. Weaning spoons should be sterilized for the first nine months. However, once your baby is crawling around and exploring objects in his mouth, there is little point in sterilizing anything other than bottles and nipples. Your baby's bowls can be washed in a dishwasher but should be wiped with a clean kitchen towel. The most popular methods of sterilizing are a microwave or steam sterilizer or tablets or solution.

Equipment

Bibs: Weaning can be a very messy business so arm yourself with a selection of bibs. Bibs with sleeves give good protection, wipe-clean bibs save on the washing, and plastic pelican bibs with a trough are suitable for older children.

Bouncy chair: A small bouncy chair that supports your baby's back is ideal for the first stages of weaning.

Ice cube trays or mini freezer containers: These allow you to prepare baby purees in bulk and freeze extra portions so that you need to cook for your baby only once or twice a week. Make sure the food is well sealed to preserve the quality.

Steamer: Steaming food is one of the best ways to preserve nutrients. A multilayered steamer is useful, as it allows you to cook several foods simultaneously.

Weaning bowls: Buy a selection of small, heatproof weaning bowls, which have suction pads on the bottom.

Weaning spoon: A baby's gums are sensitive, so instead of using a hard metal spoon, feed her with a small plastic weaning spoon. It should be shallow with no sharp edges.

Electric handheld blender: This is easy to clean and ideal for making small quantities of baby purees.

Food processor: This is good for pureeing larger quantities when making batches of purees for freezing. Many have a mini bowl attachment, which will work better with smaller quantities.

Mini processors: These are useful for making small quantities of a baby puree.

Food mill: A hand-turned food mill, such as a Mouli, is ideal for foods that have a tough skin like peas and dried apricots, as you can produce a smooth puree and hold back any indigestible husks or skins. Pureeing potato in a food processor tends to break down the starches and produces a sticky, glutinous pulp, so potato is much better pureed using a mill.

Methods of cooking

Boiling: Use the minimum amount of water and be careful not to overcook the vegetables and fruits. Add enough of the cooking liquid to make a smooth puree.

Microwaving: Chop the vegetables or fruit and put in a suitable dish. Add a little water, cover leaving an air vent, and cook on full power until tender. Puree to the desired consistency, and take care to stir well and check that it is not too hot to serve to your baby.

Steaming: This is the best way to preserve the fresh taste of and vitamins in vegetables and fruits. Vitamins B and C are water-soluble and can easily be destroyed by overcooking, especially when fruits and vegetables are boiled in water.

Freezing

You will find that if you try to make very small portions of baby purees, it will be difficult to blend them to a very smooth texture. So it is much less time consuming to prepare your baby's food in batches and freeze individual portions in ice cube trays or small freezer containers. Freeze the food as soon as it has cooled down. Baby foods can be stored in the freezer for up to six weeks.

Thaw foods either by taking them out of the freezer several hours before a meal and heating gently in a saucepan, or thaw them in a microwave. Always reheat foods thoroughly, allow to cool, and test the temperature before giving the food to your baby. If reheating in a microwave, ensure that you stir the food to get rid of any hot spots.

Never refreeze meals that have already been frozen, and do not reheat foods more than once. However, commercially frozen foods like frozen peas can be refrozen once they have been cooked.

The importance of iron

Iron is very important for your baby's physical and mental development. A baby is born with a store of iron that lasts for about the first six months. After this it is important that your baby gets the iron he needs from his diet. Iron deficiency is the most common nutritional deficiency in young children. Surveys have shown that one in every five babies aged ten to twelve months has daily intakes of iron below the recommended level. Iron deficiency can cause your child to feel tired and run down and to be more prone to infection. Between six months and two years is a critical time for brain development and a lack of iron in the diet can lead to impaired mental development.

How to spot iron deficiency

Iron deficiency can be hard to detect. Your baby may seem pale and tired; she may also seem more prone to infection. Iron deficiency may lead to anemia, which can result in irritability and loss of appetite and can impair your baby's growth and development.

Good sources of iron: *red meat, particularly liver; chicken or turkey (especially the dark meat); oily fish (canned sardines, salmon, mackerel, fresh tuna); legumes (lentils, baked beans); iron-fortified breakfast cereals; bread; egg yolk; green vegetables (spinach, broccoli); dried fruit (especially apricots).*

Tip: *Iron in foods of animal origin like red meat and poultry is much better absorbed than iron in foods of plant origin. Vitamin C also helps boost iron absorption.*

Meal planners

In this and the following chapters I have devised meal planners that will help you through weaning. Every baby develops at his own pace, so these should be used as a guide, since there are many variations on the foods that can be given and the order in which they can be introduced.

I have tried to give as wide a choice of recipes as possible, although I know that in practice, meals that your baby enjoys will be repeated many times and there is nothing wrong with giving the same food on two consecutive days—it is also a more practical proposition. Adapt the recipes according to seasonal fruits and vegetables.

First tastes: week 1

	BREAKFAST	MID-MORNING	LUNCH	MID-AFTERNOON	SUPPER	BEDTIME
DAY 1	*Breast or formula milk*	*Breast or formula milk*	*Breast or formula milk 3 teaspoons baby rice mixed with milk*	*Breast or formula milk*	*Breast or formula milk*	*Breast or formula milk*
DAY 2	*Breast or formula milk*	*Breast or formula milk*	*Breast or formula milk First Fruit Puree: apple (page 40)*	*Breast or formula milk*	*Breast or formula milk*	*Breast or formula milk*
DAY 3	*Breast or formula milk*	*Breast or formula milk*	*Breast or formula milk First Vegetable Puree: carrot (page 36)*	*Breast or formula milk*	*Breast or formula milk*	*Breast or formula milk*
DAY 4	*Breast or formula milk*	*Breast or formula milk*	*Breast or formula milk Cream of Pear Puree (page 42)*	*Breast or formula milk*	*Breast or formula milk*	*Breast or formula milk*
DAY 5	*Breast or formula milk*	*Breast or formula milk*	*Breast or formula milk First Vegetable Puree: potato or sweet potato (page 36)*	*Breast or formula milk*	*Breast or formula milk*	*Breast or formula milk*
DAY 6	*Breast or formula milk*	*Breast or formula milk*	*Breast or formula milk Apple and Pear Puree (page 42)*	*Breast or formula milk*	*Breast or formula milk*	*Breast or formula milk*
DAY 7	*Breast or formula milk*	*Breast or formula milk*	*Breast or formula milk Creamy Vegetable Puree (page 39)*	*Breast or formula milk*	*Breast or formula milk*	*Breast or formula milk*

Sugar should not be added to weaning foods except when it is necessary to improve the palatability of sour fruit.

First tastes: weeks 2 and 3

	BREAKFAST	MID-MORNING	LUNCH	MID-AFTERNOON	SUPPER	BEDTIME
DAY 1	Mashed banana	Breast or formula milk	Mixed Root Vegetable Puree (page 36)	Breast or formula milk	Breast or formula milk	Breast or formula milk
DAY 2	First Fruit Puree: apple (page 40)	Breast or formula milk	First Vegetable Puree: carrot (page 36)	Breast or formula milk	Breast or formula milk	Breast or formula milk
DAY 3	Apple and Pear Puree (page 42)	Breast or formula milk	Mixed Root Vegetable Puree (page 36)	Breast or formula milk	Breast or formula milk	Breast or formula milk
DAY 4	Cream of Pear Puree (page 42)	Breast or formula milk	Sweet Vegetable Puree (page 38)	Breast or formula milk	Breast or formula milk	Breast or formula milk
DAY 5	No-Cook Baby Food: papaya (page 40)	Breast or formula milk	First Vegetable Puree: potato or sweet potato (page 36)	Breast or formula milk	Breast or formula milk	Breast or formula milk
DAY 6	First Fruit Puree: pear (page 40)	Breast or formula milk	Creamy Vegetable Puree (page 39)	Breast or formula milk	Breast or formula milk	Breast or formula milk
DAY 7	Avocado and Banana (page 42)	Breast or formula milk	Baked Sweet Potato and Carrot Puree (page 39)	Breast or formula milk	Breast or formula milk	Breast or formula milk

Sugar should not be added to weaning foods except when it is necessary to improve the palatability of sour fruit.

First tastes: week 4 (and beyond)

	BREAKFAST	MID-MORNING	LUNCH	MID-AFTERNOON	SUPPER	BEDTIME
DAY 1	Baby cereal First Fruit Puree: apple (page 40)	Breast or formula milk	Chicken, Sweet Potato, and Pea Puree (page (57)	Breast or formula milk	Avocado and Banana (page 42)	Breast or formula milk
DAY 2	Apple, Apricot, and Pear Puree (page 46)	Breast or formula milk	Fillet of Salmon with Sweet Potato (page 62)	Breast or formula milk	Broccoli in Cheese Sauce (page 75)	Breast or formula milk
DAY 3	Banana and yogurt	Breast or formula milk	Sweet Potato and Broccoli (page 43)	Breast or formula milk	Butternut Squash and Pear (page 44)	Breast or formula milk
DAY 4	Blueberry and Pear Puree (page 46)	Breast or formula milk	Braised Beef with Carrot, Parsnip and Sweet Potato (page 44)	Breast or formula milk	Mixed Root Vegetable Puree (page 36)	Breast or formula milk
DAY 5	Apple, Apricot, and Pear Puree (page 46)	Breast or formula milk	Fruity Chicken with Butternut Squash (page 59)	Breast or formula milk	Sweet Potato and Broccoli (page 43)	Breast or formula milk
DAY 6	Dried apricots with banana puree Baby cereal	Breast or formula milk	Carrot Puree with Lentils and Cheese (page 54)	Breast or formula milk	Sweet Vegetable Puree (page 38)	Breast or formula milk
DAY 7	Banana or papaya and yogurt	Breast or formula milk	Braised Beef with Carrot, Parsnip, and Sweet Potato (page 44)	Breast or formula milk	Potato, Leek, Carrot, and Pea Puree (page 45)	Breast or formula milk

Sugar should not be added to weaning foods except when it is necessary to improve the palatability of sour fruit.

4 portions

SUPERFOODS

Carrots *are rich in beta-carotene, the plant form of vitamin A, and make excellent weaning food, as babies like their naturally sweet taste. Darker, older carrots contain more beta-carotene than baby, new carrots.*

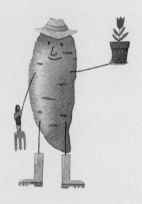

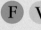 *6 portions*

SUPERFOODS

Root vegetables *make the perfect weaning food because of their naturally sweet taste and smooth texture when pureed.*

Note: *Numbers of portions for each recipe will vary depending on the age of your baby.*

First vegetable puree From 6 months

In the first few weeks of weaning, make sure that carrots are cooked for quite a long time so that they are soft enough to puree to a smooth consistency. This method for cooking carrots also works with any of the other root vegetables, such as potatoes, sweet potatoes, and rutabagas. Cooking times will differ depending on which vegetable you choose.

4 medium carrots

Wash and peel the carrots and chop or slice into even-size pieces. Put in a steamer or colander set over boiling water and cook until tender (15 to 20 minutes). Alternatively, put the vegetables in a saucepan and pour in just enough boiling water to cover. Cover and simmer until soft (15 to 20 minutes).

Puree until very smooth together with some of the cooking liquid or some of the water in the bottom of the steamer. The amount of liquid you add really depends on your baby; you may need to add a little more if your baby finds it difficult to swallow.

To microwave, place the carrots in a suitable dish. Add 3 tablespoons cooled boiled water and cover with microwave-safe plastic wrap. Pierce a few times and cook on high for 9 to 10 minutes, stirring halfway through the cooking time. Blend to a puree, adding some extra cooled boiled water to make a smooth consistency.

Spoon some of the puree into your baby's bowl and serve lukewarm.

Mixed root vegetable puree From 6 months

Mix and match a selection of three root vegetables. Use approximately half a pound of each but less of the parsnip, as it has quite a strong taste. Choose from the vegetables below.

carrot / potato / sweet potato / butternut squash / rutabaga / parsnip

Wash, peel, and chop your chosen vegetables, place them in a saucepan, and just cover with boiling water. Cook over medium heat until tender (about 20 minutes). Blend the vegetables to a smooth puree using as much of the cooking liquid as necessary. Alternatively, steam the vegetables until tender, blending to a puree using some of the boiled water from the bottom of the steamer. You can also add some of your baby's usual milk as well as some of the cooking liquid. Spoon some of the puree into your baby's bowl and serve lukewarm.

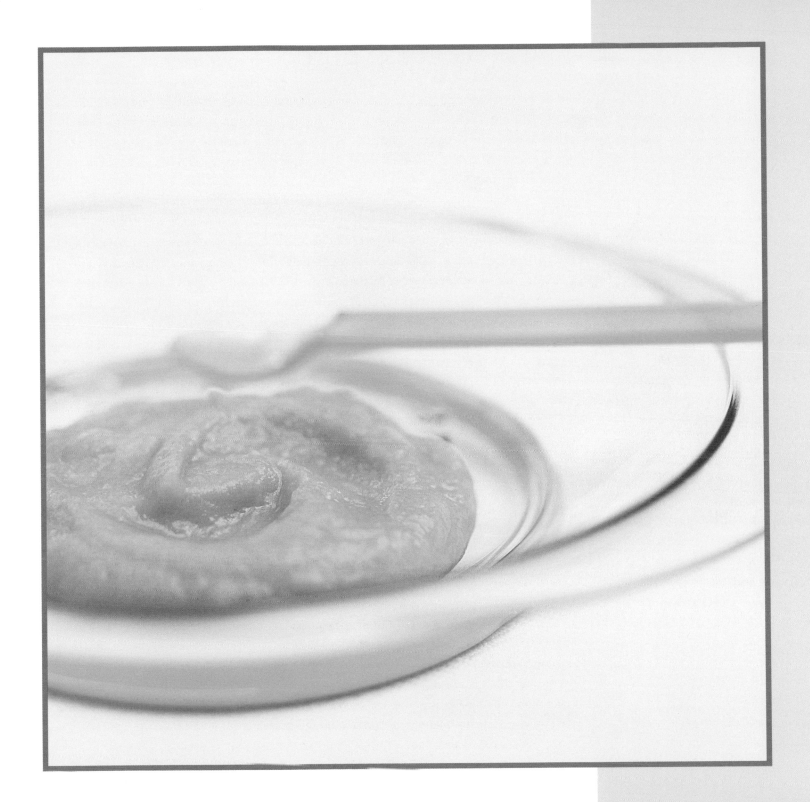

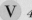
SUPERFOODS

Butternut squash

is easily digested and rarely causes allergies; therefore it makes perfect weaning food.

  2 portions

SUPERFOODS

Parsnips *provide a good source of starch and fiber. They also contain the anti-oxidant vitamins C and E.*

Sweet vegetable puree From 6 months

All of the vegetables in these recipes are readily available in supermarkets and can be made into delicious purees for your baby. The naturally sweet taste of butternut squash tends to be very popular with babies.

1 large butternut squash

Peel and seed the squash, then cut into small pieces. Place in a steamer and cook until tender (about 15 minutes). Alternatively, place in a pan with a little water, cover, and simmer until tender. Drain and blend to a puree, adding a little of the cooking water if necessary.

Butternut squash can also be baked in the oven. Preheat the oven to 350°F. Cut the squash in half, scoop out the seeds, and brush with some melted unsalted butter. Cover with foil and bake in the oven until tender (about 1¼ hours).

To microwave, peel and dice the squash. Place in a suitable microwave dish and sprinkle with 3 tablespoons water. Cover with microwave-safe plastic wrap, pierce, and cook on high for 7 to 8 minutes, stirring halfway through. Let stand, covered, for 4 minutes. Puree and then spoon some of the puree into your baby's bowl and serve lukewarm.

Parsnip or carrot and apple puree From 6 months

Fruit and vegetable combinations work well together. Also try apple and carrot.

1 medium parsnip or 2 medium carrots
1 small apple

Scrub, trim, and peel the parsnip or carrots and cut into chunks. Place the chunks in a steamer and cover and cook for 15 minutes. Peel, core, and chop the apple, add to the parsnip or carrot, and continue cooking for another 5 minutes. Drain and puree to a smooth consistency, adding a little of the water from the bottom of the steamer if necessary. Spoon some of the puree into your baby's bowl and serve lukewarm.

Baked sweet potato and carrot puree From 6 months

Baking sweet potatoes in the oven enhances their naturally sweet taste, so this is a good puree to make if you are making a roast for the rest of the family, as you can just pop the sweet potato into the oven to cook alongside. It is also very tasty without the added carrot.

1 medium sweet potato
2 medium carrots, peeled and sliced
2 to 3 tablespoons your baby's usual milk

Preheat the oven to 375°F. Wash and dry the sweet potato and prick all over with a fork. Bake in the oven until tender (about 45 minutes). Meanwhile, steam or boil the carrots until tender (about 20 minutes). When the sweet potato is soft, allow to cool down a little, then cut it in half and scoop out the flesh. Puree together with the cooked carrot and the milk.

Alternatively, you can cook the sweet potato in a microwave. Pierce several holes in the potato with a fork. Place on at least two layers of microwave-safe paper towels. Microwave on high for 5 minutes, turning halfway through the cooking time. Let stand for 5 minutes. Peel and puree with the carrot and a little of your baby's usual milk.

Creamy vegetable puree From 6 months

Stronger-tasting vegetables such as parsnip, carrot, and broccoli can be given a more creamy mild taste by combining them with some baby rice and milk.

1 tablespoon baby rice cereal
3 tablespoons your baby's usual milk
¼ cup vegetable puree

Mix the baby rice and milk together according to the package instructions and stir into the vegetable puree until thoroughly combined.

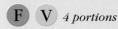 **F** **V** *4 portions*

Sweet potato *comes in two varieties: orange-fleshed and creamy-fleshed. Both have red skins and both are good sources of potassium, vitamin C, and fiber. However, I prefer to use the orange-fleshed variety, which is also an excellent source of beta-carotene. This helps to prevent certain types of cancer and mops up free radicals.*

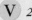 **F** **V** *2 portions*

Baby rice *should be the first cereal you introduce because it does not contain gluten, a protein found in wheat, oats, barley, and rye that can cause food allergy if introduced before six months.*

SUPERFOODS

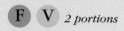
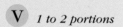
First fruit puree From 6 months

Choose only sweet ripe fruit for your baby. Some apples like Granny Smith can have quite a tart flavor and are not as sweet as other varieties.

2 medium apples or 2 ripe pears, peeled and cored
2 tablespoons water or unsweetened apple juice

Chop the apple or pear into small, even-size pieces. Put the fruit into a heavy-bottomed saucepan with the water, cover, and cook over low heat until tender (6 to 8 minutes for apples, about 4 minutes for pears).

To microwave, chop the apple or pear into small, even-size pieces. Place the fruit in a suitable dish, add 2 to 3 tablespoons water, and cover with microwave-safe plastic wrap. Pierce several times and then cook on full power until the fruit is tender (about 2 minutes).

Blend the fruit to a smooth puree using some of the cooking liquid. Spoon a little puree into your baby's bowl and serve lukewarm.

No-cook baby food From 6 months

Some mothers say that they just don't have the time to make their own baby food, but there is nothing better for your baby than good-quality fresh food. Here are some ideas for making delicious and nutritious baby food in minutes. So now there's no excuse! Always choose ripe fruit and serve at once.

Papaya
Cut a small papaya in half, remove the black seeds, and puree or mash the flesh of one half until smooth.

Avocado
Cut a small avocado in half, remove the pit, scoop out the flesh of one half, and mash together with a little of your baby's usual milk.

Banana
Mash the banana with a fork. During the first stages of weaning add a little milk if necessary to thin down the consistency and add a familiar taste.

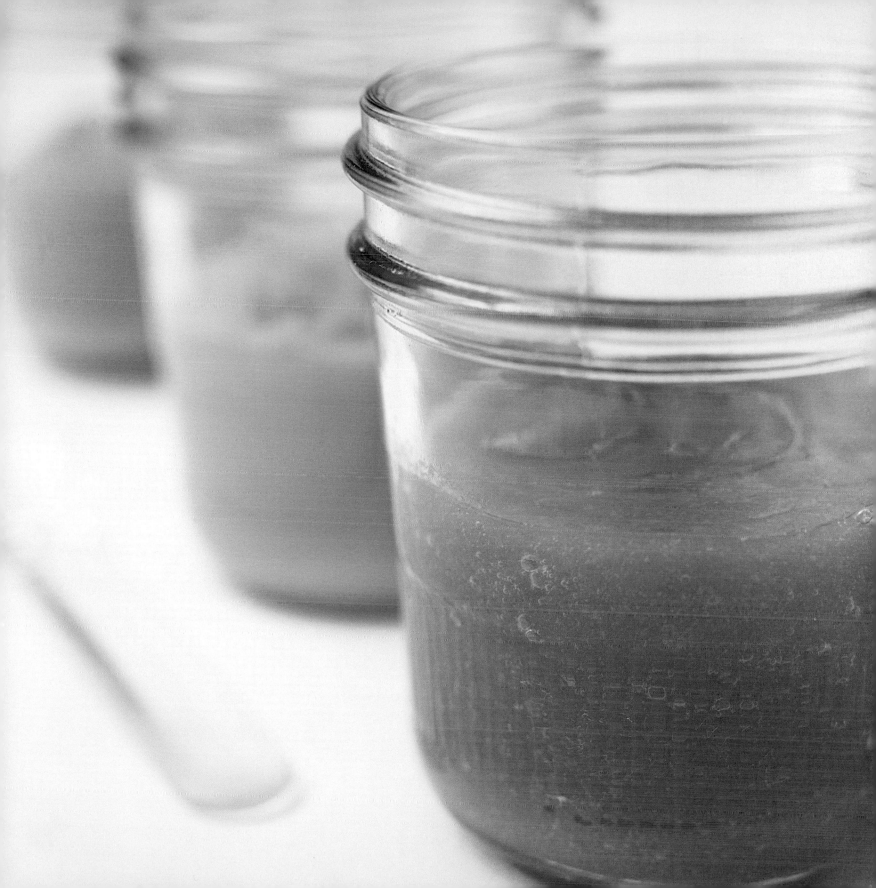

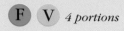
SUPERFOODS

Pears *are one of the least allergenic foods, so they make great weaning food.*

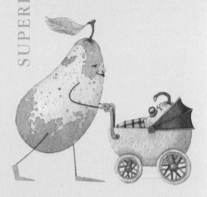

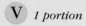 *1 portion*

SUPERFOODS

Bananas *are full of slow-release sugars, which provide sustained energy. They make perfect portable baby food, as they come in their own easy-to-peel packaging. They are also good for the treatment of diarrhea and constipation.*

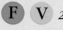 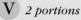 *2 portions*

SUPERFOODS

Baby rice *is gluten free, is easily digested, and has a milky taste that helps to ease your baby's transition from a purely milk-based diet to solids. It is a good thickener for runny purees like pear, peach, and plum.*

Apple and pear puree From 6 months

Apple and pear blend well together. You could add a small cinnamon stick to introduce a new flavor. Simply remove the stick before pureeing the fruit or add a pinch of ground cinnamon when cooking. Choose sweet apples like Gala.

2 apples, peeled, cored, and chopped
2 pears, peeled, cored, and chopped
¼ cup unsweetened apple juice or water
2 tablespoons water

Put the fruit into a heavy-bottomed saucepan with the apple juice and 2 tablespoons water, cover, and cook over low heat until tender (6 to 8 minutes). Blend the fruit to a smooth puree. Spoon a little puree into your baby's bowl and serve lukewarm.

Avocado and banana From 6 months

¼ avocado
½ small banana
1 to 2 tablespoons your baby's usual milk

Mash the avocado together with the banana and the milk. You can substitute the flesh of half a small papaya for the banana in this recipe. If using papaya, the milk is then optional.

Cream of pear puree From 6 months

2 small pears, peeled, cored, and cut into chunks
1 tablespoon baby rice cereal
1 tablespoon your baby's usual milk

Put the pear into a small saucepan and cover and cook for 2 to 3 minutes. Blend to a smooth puree. Mix together the baby rice and milk and stir this into the pear puree.

Vegetables at 6 months after first tastes accepted

Naturally sweet-tasting root vegetable purees are easy to digest and are ideal for early weaning. But after a few weeks you can introduce stronger-tasting vegetables like broccoli.

Zucchini

Zucchini is best mixed with another vegetable and it goes well with sweet potato, carrot, pumpkin, potato, and rutabaga. Wash, trim, and slice a medium zucchini. Place in a steamer and cook until tender (10 to 12 minutes). Alternatively, place in a pan with a little boiling water. Cover and simmer gently until tender (6 to 8 minutes).

To microwave, place the zucchini slices in a microwaveable dish and add 1 tablespoon water. Cover with microwave-safe plastic wrap, pierce the wrap, and microwave on high until tender (about 6 minutes). Stir halfway through. Let stand for 3 minutes before turning into a puree.

Cauliflower or broccoli

Place about 2 cups small cauliflower or broccoli florets in a steamer and cook until tender (about 10 minutes). Drain and blend to a puree with a little of the boiled water from the steamer. Alternatively, add just enough boiling water to cover the vegetables, then cover and simmer until tender (about 10 minutes).

To microwave, place the florets in a microwaveable dish, sprinkle with 2 tablespoons water, and cover with microwave-safe plastic wrap. Pierce the wrap and microwave on high until tender (about 6 minutes), stirring halfway through. Let stand for 4 minutes, then blend with a little of your baby's usual milk or boiled water to make a smooth puree. Broccoli has quite a strong taste and is best mixed with potato, sweet potato, pumpkin, or rutabaga or a cheese sauce (see page 75).

Sweet potato and broccoli From 6 months

1 medium sweet potato, peeled and diced
3 broccoli florets

Steam the vegetables until tender (sweet potato: about 12 minutes; broccoli: 7 to 8 minutes). Puree together with a little of the water from the bottom of the steamer. Spoon some of the puree into your baby's bowl and serve lukewarm.

  4 portions

Zucchini *is a good source of beta-carotene, but most of the nutrients lie in the skin, so do not peel it.*

Broccoli *is a true SuperFood, as it is a great source of vitamin C and also contains beta-carotene, folic acid, iron, potassium, and anticancer phytonutrients.*

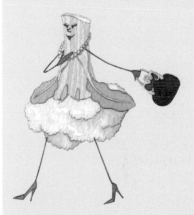

  3 portions

Broccoli *is best steamed or microwaved, as boiling it in water halves its vitamin C content. If your baby isn't keen on the taste, mix it with a sweet-tasting vegetable like sweet potato, rutabaga, or butternut squash.*

SUPERFOODS

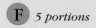
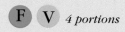
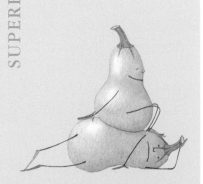

Braised beef with carrot, parsnip, and sweet potato From 6 months

This recipe makes a good introduction to red meat. The root vegetables give the meat a smooth texture and a flavor that babies like. You can also introduce chicken to your baby once first tastes are accepted.

1 tablespoon olive oil
1 small red onion, chopped
1 clove garlic, crushed
4$\frac{1}{2}$ ounces lean beef, cut into pieces
2 tablespoons all-purpose flour
2 medium carrots, peeled and sliced

1 small parsnip, peeled and sliced
1 medium sweet potato,
   peeled and chopped
1 bay leaf
1 tablespoon chopped fresh parsley
1$\frac{1}{2}$ cups unsalted chicken stock

Heat the olive oil in a heavy-bottomed saucepan or small casserole. Sauté the onion and garlic for 3 to 4 minutes or until softened. Toss the pieces of beef in the flour and sauté until sealed. Add the carrots, parsnip, sweet potato, bay leaf, and parsley to the pan and pour in the stock. Bring to a boil and then simmer for about 1 hour 45 minutes or until the meat is tender. Blend, adding as much of the cooking liquid as necessary.

Butternut squash and pear From 6 months

The naturally sweet taste of butternut squash is generally very popular with babies, and it combines very well with a variety of fruits. Try also butternut squash and peach when ripe, juicy peaches are in season.

1 large butternut squash, peeled, seeded, and chopped
1 juicy pear, peeled, cored, and chopped

Steam the butternut squash until tender (about 12 minutes). Add the pear and continue to steam for about 3 minutes. Puree with about 2 tablespoons of the water from the bottom of the steamer. You can also cut the butternut squash in half, brush with melted butter, cover loosely with foil, and bake in the oven at 350ºF for 1 hour or until tender.

Potato, leek, carrot, and pea puree

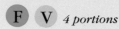 4 portions

2 tablespoons unsalted butter

⅓ cup washed and sliced white part of a leek

1 large potato, peeled and diced

1 medium carrot, peeled and sliced

1¼ cups unsalted chicken stock or vegetable stock

⅔ cup frozen peas

Melt the butter in a saucepan and sauté the leek for 3 to 4 minutes. Add the potato and carrot and pour in the stock. Bring to a boil, then reduce the heat, cover, and cook for 10 minutes. Add the peas and continue to cook until the vegetables are tender (about 6 minutes). Puree in a food processor.

Fruits at 6 months after first tastes accepted

Naturally fruits can be pureed on their own or mixed with a little baby rice, banana, or pear. Make sure that you choose fruit that is sweet and ripe.

Peaches and nectarines

Score a cross on the base of the fruit, then submerge in boiling water for 1 minute. Drain, peel, and chop the peach or nectarine, discarding the pit, and then puree.

Plums and apricots

Choose sweet ripe plums or apricots. Peel by submerging the fruit in boiling water (see above) and cut into quarters and discard the pits. Steam for a few minutes until soft and then puree. Both plums and apricots combine well with pureed apple.

Melons

Scoop out and discard the seeds from a small wedge of melon. Remove the skin and cut the flesh into chunks. Puree until smooth. Melon is also good with mashed banana or avocado.

Dried apricots and peaches

Simmer dried apricots in water until soft, then puree in a food mill to get rid of the tough skins and add a little of the cooking liquid to make a smooth puree. Dried apricot puree is good mixed with baby rice and milk, or mashed banana or apple or pear puree.

SUPERFOODS

Potatoes *contain vitamin C and are a good source of potassium. They also blend well with most vegetables.*

Healthy eating:

Peel potatoes just before cooking. Don't soak in water, as they will then lose their vitamin C.

SUPERFOODS

Peaches *provide a good source of vitamin C, and the soft flesh is easy to digest.*

Apricots *are a good source of beta-carotene and also contain fiber.*

Cantaloupe *is the most nutritious variety of melon. It is very sweet and rich in vitamin C and beta-carotene.*

Dried apricots *are a great source of beta-carotene and are a good source of iron and potassium. The drying process increases their concentration. (See preservative warning on page 46.)*

1 to 2 portions

Blueberries *are rich in vitamin C and also contain beta-carotene. The blue pigment anthocyanin in the skin of the blueberries helps protect us against cancer. Blueberries have the highest antioxidant capacity of all fruits, mainly because of the anthocyanin in their skin.*

  2 portions

Dried apricots *are one of nature's great health foods. It is best to choose moist apricots, as they are nice and soft, but make sure they have not been treated with sulfur dioxide before drying in order to preserve the bright orange color and to prevent fungal growth. This substance can trigger an asthma attack in susceptible babies.*

Dried fruits are rich in potassium, which helps counteract the high salt content of fast foods like burgers and fries. Dried apricots make a good high-energy snack.

Blueberry and pear puree From 6 months

This is a quick and easy puree to make, and the blueberries turn it a wonderful deep purple. Berry fruits can sometimes cause reactions in allergic young babies, so don't give them to your baby if there is any sign of a reaction and consult your doctor for advice.

1 large juicy pear, peeled, cored, and chopped
¼ cup blueberries
1½ teaspoons baby rice cereal

Put the fruit into a saucepan and simmer for about 5 minutes. Puree and stir in the baby rice cereal. Spoon some of the puree into your baby's bowl and serve lukewarm.

Apple, apricot, and pear puree From 6 months

This makes a delicious and nutritious combination of fruits. It can be mixed either with baby rice, as in the recipe below, or with mashed banana. Banana, however, cannot be frozen, so freeze the puree in individual containers without the baby rice and add the rice or mashed banana just before serving, once you have thawed and reheated your baby's meal.

1 apple, peeled, cored, and chopped
8 dried apricots, roughly chopped
1 pear, peeled, cored, and chopped
1 tablespoon baby rice cereal
2 tablespoons your baby's usual milk

Place the apple and dried apricots in a saucepan with ¼ cup water. Cover and simmer for 5 minutes. Add the pear and continue to simmer for 2 minutes. Puree the fruit until smooth. In a small bowl, mix the baby rice cereal with the milk until smooth and stir into the fruit puree.

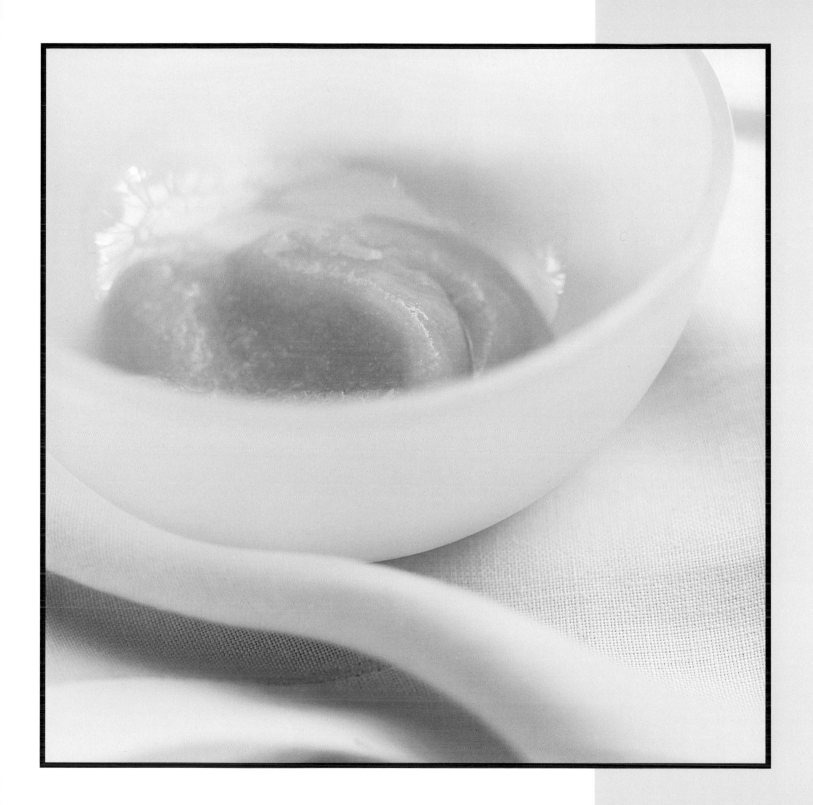

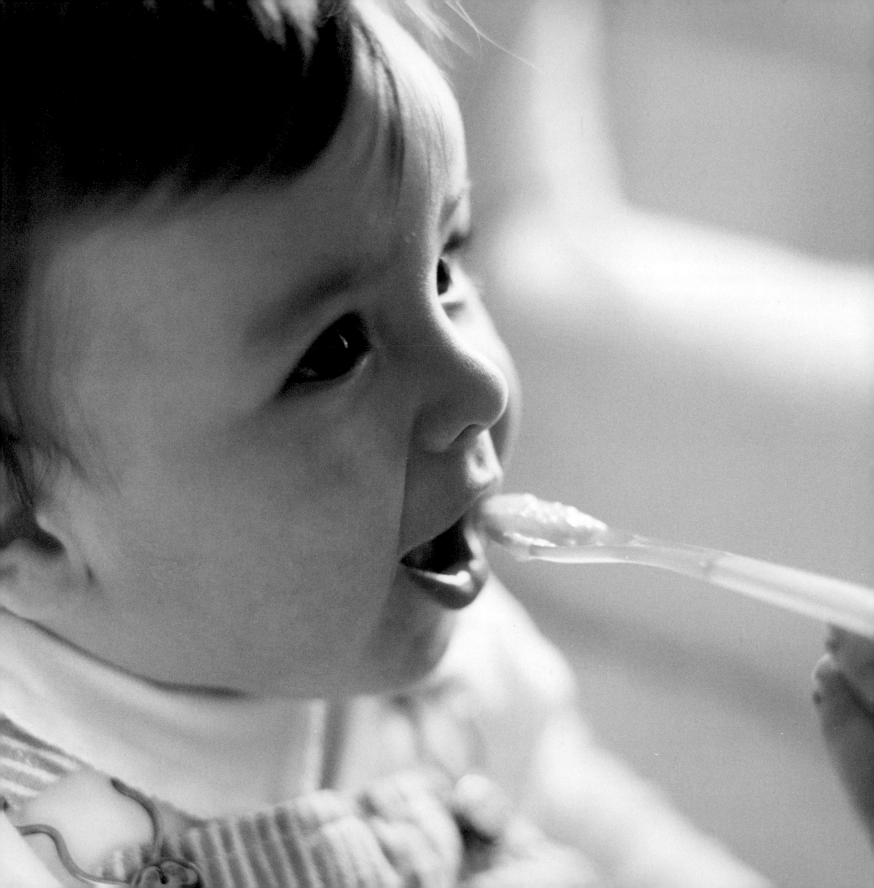

7 to 9 months:

exploring new tastes and textures

Babies develop rapidly between seven and nine months, and your baby will soon be sitting in a high chair. She will be ready for stronger tastes and more challenging textures.

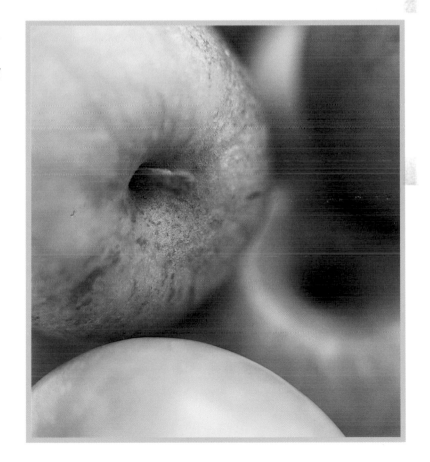

The next hurdles

By the age of seven months, your baby should be eating three meals a day. The quantity will vary from child to child, but by this stage your baby is ready to enjoy a wide variety of tastes. This is a stage of quite rapid development and your baby will spend many more hours awake. Whereas a six-month-old baby still needs to be supported when you are feeding him, a nine-month-old is usually strong enough to sit in a high chair.

Try to make eating a sociable event and let your baby join you at mealtimes whenever possible. Never force a baby to eat something he doesn't want. Instead, let your baby's appetite be your guide. As long as your baby is happy and continues to grow, he should be fine.

Babies should have 18 to 20 ounces of formula or breast milk each day up to the age of one year. A portion of the milk intake can come from dairy products like cheese and yogurt. If your baby is not hungry at mealtimes, you may find that cutting down on the amount of milk your baby drinks will mean that he is hungrier for his solids and therefore not so fussy about the texture of his food.

Introducing more texture

Having introduced a wide range of single ingredient purees, you can now combine foods to make tasty meals for your baby. As teeth begin to emerge (see page 52), introduce slightly coarser textures into your baby's food and soft finger foods. Your baby will probably still mostly use his gums to chew and it is surprising how efficient these are at chomping their way through food. It is not a good idea to continue giving only smooth purees for too long or your baby may become lazy about chewing and have difficulty developing the tongue movement needed to cope with solids.

New foods to introduce

At this age, babies should eat foods each day from each of the food groups: starches, fruit and vegetables, dairy, and protein (see pages 13 and 14).

- *Wheat-based foods such as pasta and bread.*
- *Low-sugar cereals like unflavored oatmeal and shredded wheat. Avoid large amounts of high-fiber foods like bran, as these are difficult for babies to digest and can deplete the body of vital nutrients.*
- *Dairy products such as cheese and yogurt made with whole milk. Low-fat dairy products such as low-fat yogurt are not suitable, as they are too low in calories for growing babies. Avoid soft cheeses like Camembert and Brie because of the risk of listeriosis.*
- *Cow's milk is low in iron and vitamin D, so babies should continue with breast or formula milk for the first year. However, cow's milk can be used in cooking or with your baby's cereal.*
- *Lean red meat and poultry.*
- *Mild-tasting fish such as flounder, cod, and salmon. Many children grow up disliking fish, which is a great shame, so I try very hard to come up with really tasty fish recipes.*
- *Stronger-flavored vegetables such as leeks, spinach, onions, and mushrooms. At 8 or 9 months try steamed vegetables like carrot sticks or broccoli florets.*
- *Citrus fruits.*
- *Berry fruits (strain to get rid of the seeds).*
- *Stronger-tasting fruits such as mango.*
- *Lentils and split peas.*
- *Tofu.*
- *Eggs: hard-boiled or well cooked, such as in an omelet.*

For a gradual introduction you could mix some mashed or grated food with some of your baby's favorite purees. Don't expect him to be thrilled by this change, as lumps take a bit of getting used to. Some babies will cope very well with chopped food at nine months, but others still prefer smoother textures.

Another way to introduce texture into your baby's meals is to prepare a fairly smooth puree and then add some tiny cooked pasta shapes. For older children you can mix cooked pasta shapes with bite-size pieces of cooked vegetables like carrots, green beans, and broccoli. Chewing and swallowing lumpy food is linked to speech development. Some babies prefer finger foods that melt in the mouth, like banana, peach, or fingers of toast, to lumpy food.

Learning to eat red meat

I think that sometimes we mistakenly believe that babies don't like the taste of certain foods when, in fact, it is the texture that they object to. This is often the case with meat. Unless you choose to bring up your child as a vegetarian, red meat is an excellent food, as it provides the best source of iron, which is vitally important for both physical and mental development. Babies are born with a store of iron that lasts for about six months. After this it is important to make sure they get the iron they need from their food. A baby's iron requirements are particularly high between six and twelve months.

The trouble is that meat can be very chewy, and so I have found that the best way to make it more palatable is to combine it with root vegetables or pasta, both of which will help to produce a much smoother and easier to swallow texture. I find that

when cooking ground meat for older babies—for example, as a Bolognese sauce—it is still much better received if once the meat is cooked, it is then chopped for a few seconds in a food processor.

Self-feeding

Let your baby experiment with feeding herself, using her fingers or a spoon. The more independent your growing baby, the sooner she will master the art of feeding herself. See page 70 for suitable finger foods.

Equipment

High chair: Once your baby can support her head and upper body, she can use a high chair. But if your baby is active, don't put her there until her meal is ready in case she gets upset at being confined to one place for too long. Put her in a safety harness so that she can't wriggle and fall out. Meals are not just about nutrition, they are a time for being sociable, so let her join in with family meals by pulling the high chair up to the table.

Bowls and spoons: A plastic bowl with a suction pad on the base is a good idea at this age; throwing food on the floor is often as much fun as eating it. As soon as you think she is ready, give her a plastic spoon and fork: She can experiment with feeding herself. Getting food onto a spoon is easier if the food is in a bowl rather than on a plate.

Feeding cups: Many babies can learn to drink from a feeding cup around the age of six months. Start with a double-handled cup with a soft spout and snap-tight lid. There are many varieties, including no-spill cups and cups with a one-way valve control so that even if the cup is turned upside down, no liquid will come out. Eventually graduate to an open cup.

Your baby's first teeth

Your baby will be teething from around six to eighteen months and so gums may be sore and your child may be quite unsettled and not interested in food. A chilled teething ring can help soothe sore gums. You could also give chilled raw vegetables like sticks of carrot or cucumber. Rubbing an infant teething gel onto the gums may help—they contain local anesthetics and can be prescribed by a pediatrician, who is the best person to decide whether they are suitable or not.

Teeth begin to erupt from six months onward, and four to eight teeth are usually present by the age of twelve months. You should start brushing your baby's teeth as soon as the first one appears. Brush your child's teeth thoroughly twice a day, using a small, pea-size blob of children's toothpaste on a small baby toothbrush with soft fibers. Do not put a lot of toothpaste on your child's toothbrush, particularly in areas where fluoride is already added to tap water. Too much fluoride can cause dental fluorosis, which can permanently discolor children's teeth. Alternatively, you could wrap a clean cotton cloth around your finger and gently rub the teeth and gums.

Ways to prevent cavities

- *Use a cup as soon as your child is able to hold one.*
- *Diluted juice with meals is fine, but it is best to give water or milk between meals.*
- *Do not put your child to bed with a bottle.*
- *Do not use bottles to feed juice or as comforters.*
- *Do not bottle-feed after one year of age.*

Baby bottle tooth decay

Drinking from a bottle is worse for teeth than drinking from a cup because the milk or juice is in contact with the teeth for longer. Nursing bottle cavities, also known as baby bottle tooth decay, occurs when a young baby or small child is frequently given sugary drinks in a bottle. The bacteria present on teeth use sugar to produce acid, which attacks tooth enamel and leads to tooth decay. It is even worse to give a baby a bottle to suck at night when there is less saliva than usual, which results in sugar clinging to the teeth. It is much better to give water between meals, reserving fruit juice for mealtimes only. If your child insists on a bottle to take to bed, then use water. It is a good idea to start using a lidded cup with a spout from the age of six or seven months and eventually move on to a cup. Try to dispense with bottles by the time your baby is one year old (see also page 68).

Tooth-friendly snacks

- Vegetable sticks on their own or with a dip.
- Cheese or cheese on toast.
- Sugar-free teething biscuits or zwiebacks.
- Fingers of toast or bagels.
- Cream cheese with mini bread sticks, rice cakes, or oatcakes.
- Mini sandwiches with peanut butter or egg salad.
- A bowl of homemade soup or fresh soup from a carton.
- Mini salads, such as mozzarella and tomato, pasta, tuna, and corn.
- Fresh fruit. Biting on frozen fruit can help numb the pain of teething.

Healthy eating: *Teething often causes your baby to drool, so it is a good idea to put a little petroleum jelly around your baby's mouth and chin to help prevent the area from becoming dry and red.*

Meal planner

Vary the desserts with lunch and supper. Give your baby some fresh fruit like a banana or grated apple, fruit puree, and occasionally other desserts like ice cream, rice pudding, and fruit yogurt.

	BREAKFAST	MID-MORNING	LUNCH	MID-AFTERNOON	SUPPER	BEDTIME
DAY 1	*Breast or formula milk* My Favorite Oatmeal (page 65) Fruit	*Breast or formula milk*	Chicken, Sweet Potato, and Pea Puree (page 57)	*Breast or formula milk*	Vegetable Puree with Tomato and Cheese (page 62)	*Breast or formula milk*
DAY 2	*Breast or formula milk* Cereal Banana	*Breast or formula milk*	My First Fish Puree (page 61)	*Breast or formula milk*	Eat Your Greens Puree (page 57)	*Breast or formula milk*
DAY 3	*Breast or formula milk* Apricot, Papaya, and Tofu with baby rice and milk (page 64)	*Breast or formula milk*	My First Chicken Puree (page 59)	*Breast or formula milk*	Carrot Puree with Lentils and Cheese (page 54)	*Breast or formula milk*
DAY 4	*Breast or formula milk* Cheese on toast Strawberry, Peach, and Apple Puree (page 64)	*Breast or formula milk*	Old-fashioned Beef Casserole (page 60)	*Breast or formula milk*	Parsnip or Carrot and Apple Puree (page 38)	*Breast or formula milk*
DAY 5	*Breast or formula milk* Cereal and yogurt	*Breast or formula milk*	Fruity Chicken with Butternut Squash (page 59)	*Breast or formula milk*	Tasty Trio of Root Vegetables (page 54)	*Breast or formula milk*
DAY 6	*Breast or formula milk* Well-cooked scrambled egg with fingers of toast	*Breast or formula milk*	Fillet of Salmon with Sweet Potato (page 62)	*Breast or formula milk*	Chicken, Sweet Potato, and Pea Puree (page 57)	*Breast or formula milk*
DAY 7	*Breast or formula milk* Apple, Pear, and Prune with Oats (page 65) Raisin toast fingers	*Breast or formula milk*	Chicken, Sweet Potato, and Pea Puree (page 57)	*Breast or formula milk*	Vegetable Puree with Tomato and Cheese (page 62) Fingers of toast	*Breast or formula milk*

Lentils *are a good source of protein and fiber. They are also a rich source of potassium, zinc, and folic acid. Both cheese and lentils are good nutrient-dense foods for growing babies.*

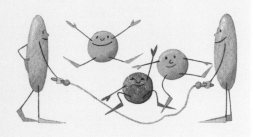

F V *6 portions*

Sweet potatoes *are rich in vitamins C and E and beta-carotene, so sometimes it's a good idea to substitute them for ordinary potatoes.*

Healthy eating:

Frozen vegetables for baby purees can be just as nutritious as fresh.

Carrot puree with lentils and cheese

½ cup finely chopped onion
1½ teaspoons vegetable oil
2 tablespoons red lentils
3 medium carrots, peeled and sliced
1½ cups boiling water
1 tablespoon unsalted butter
2 tomatoes, peeled, seeded, and roughly chopped
½ cup grated Cheddar cheese

In a saucepan, sauté the onion in the vegetable oil until softened (3 to 4 minutes). Rinse the lentils and drain and add to the onion. Add the carrots and pour in the boiling water. Bring to a boil, then cover the saucepan and cook over medium heat for 25 minutes. Melt the butter in a saucepan and sauté the tomatoes until mushy, then stir in the Cheddar cheese.

Drain the carrot and lentil mixture and reserve the cooking liquid. Combine the carrots and lentils together with ½ cup of the cooking liquid and the tomato and cheese mixture in a food processor and puree to a smooth consistency.

Tasty trio of root vegetables

The orange-fleshed sweet potato is richer in nutrients than the white-fleshed sweet potato. You can buy unsalted vegetable bouillon cubes from a supermarket.

2 tablespoons unsalted butter
⅓ cup washed and sliced white part of a leek
1 large sweet potato, peeled and diced
1 medium carrot, peeled and sliced
1 small parsnip, peeled and diced
1½ cups unsalted vegetable stock

Melt the butter in a saucepan and sauté the leek for 3 to 4 minutes. Add the sweet potato, carrots, and parsnip, pour in the stock, bring to a boil, and then cover and simmer for 20 minutes. Puree in a food processor or mash for older babies.

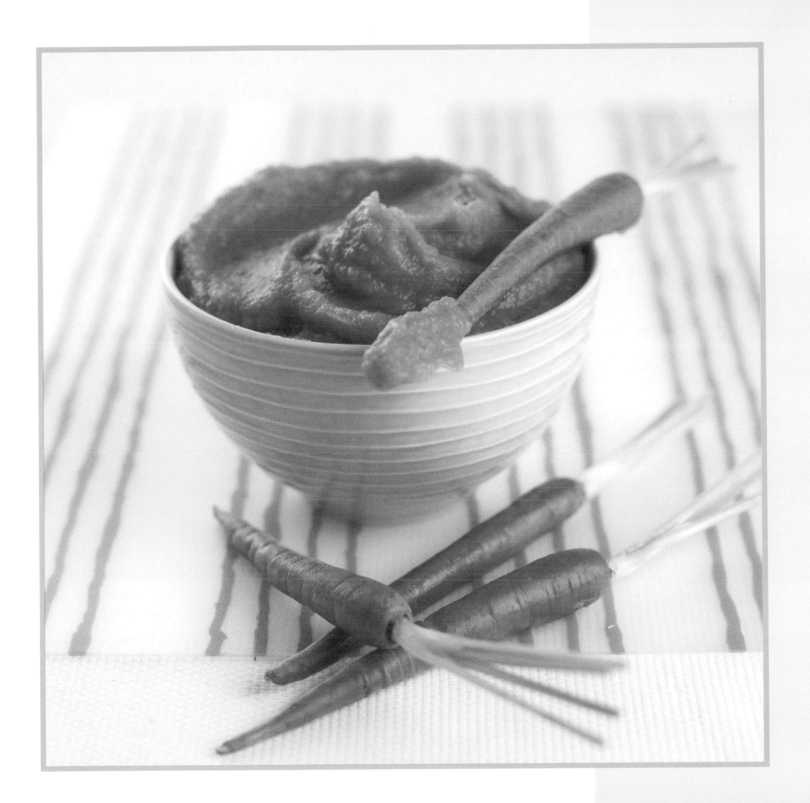

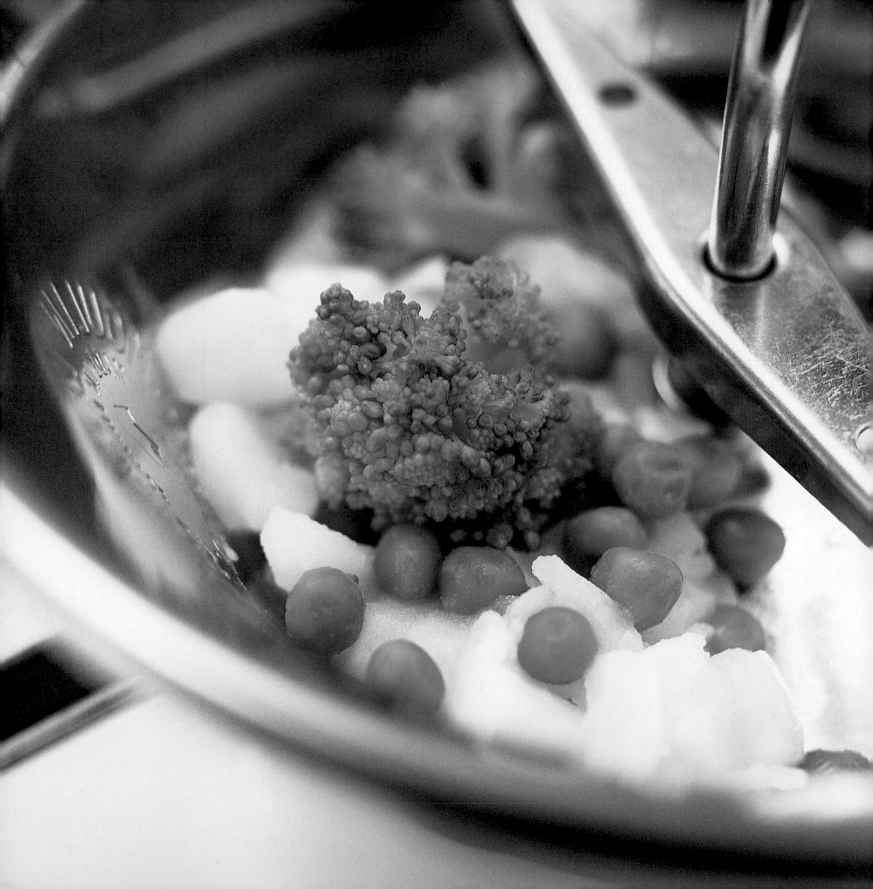

Chicken, sweet potato, and pea puree

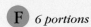 **F** *6 portions*

Not only does this taste delicious, but it is also packed full of vitamins, since both sweet potatoes and carrots are excellent sources of vitamin A. The naturally sweet taste and smooth texture of sweet potato makes this an ideal puree for introducing young babies to their first taste of chicken.

1 tablespoon vegetable oil

½ small onion, chopped

4 ounces boneless, skinless chicken breast, cut into pieces

1 large sweet potato, peeled and diced

1 medium carrot, peeled and sliced

1¼ cups unsalted chicken stock

1 cup frozen peas

Heat the vegetable oil in a saucepan and sauté the onion for 2 to 3 minutes. Add the chicken and sauté until sealed. Add the sweet potato and carrot and pour in the chicken stock. Bring to a boil, then cover and simmer for 20 minutes. Add the frozen peas and continue to cook for an additional 5 minutes. Puree in a food processor.

Eat your greens puree

 F **V** *4 portions*

It's a good idea to introduce your baby to the flavor of green vegetables early on. However, sometimes babies find the taste of some vegetables too strong, so it can be a good idea to mix stronger-tasting vegetables like broccoli together with potato. You could also make this puree using other green vegetables like spinach or zucchini.

⅓ cup chopped onion

1 tablespoon unsalted butter

3 medium potatoes, peeled and diced

1½ cups unsalted vegetable stock or water

½ cup chopped broccoli florets

⅔ cup frozen peas

Sauté the onion in the butter until softened but not colored (about 5 minutes). Add the potatoes, pour in the stock or water, cover, bring to a boil, and cook for 10 minutes. Add the broccoli and cook for 3 minutes. Then add the peas and cook for an additional 3 minutes. Puree in a food mill.

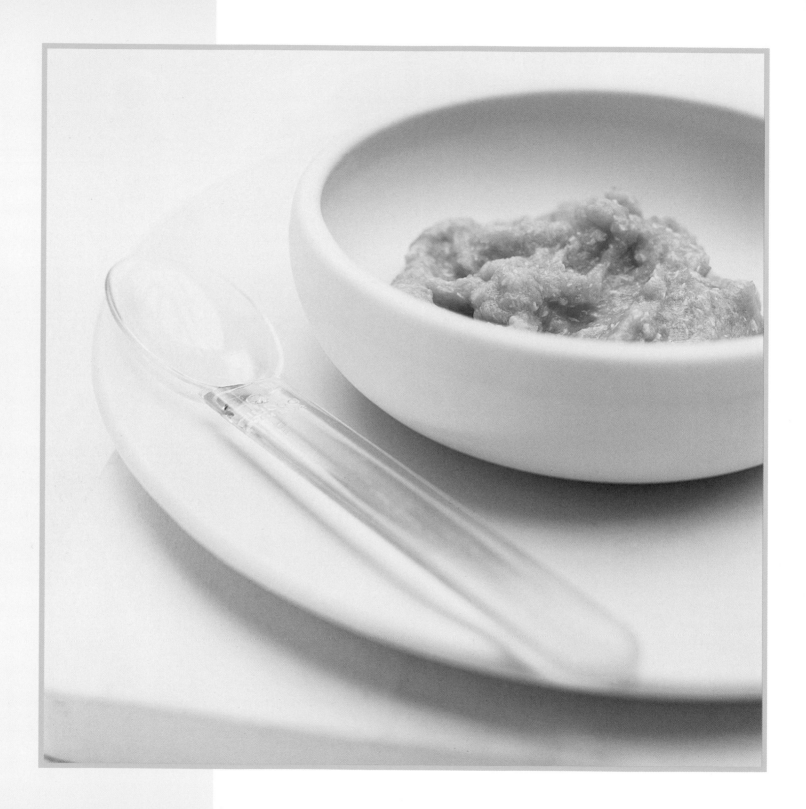

My first chicken puree

Chicken blends well with many vegetables, and mixing it with root vegetables helps to give this puree a smooth texture to make a good introduction to chicken.

¼ cup washed and sliced white part of a leek
1 tablespoon vegetable oil
3 ounces boneless, skinless chicken breast,
   cut into chunks
2 medium potatoes, peeled and diced

2 medium carrots, peeled and sliced
2 plum tomatoes, peeled, seeded,
   and chopped
1 cup unsalted chicken stock

Sauté the leek in the vegetable oil until softened (about 3 minutes). Then add the chicken and sauté until it has sealed. Add the potatoes, carrots, and tomatoes and pour in the chicken stock. Bring to a boil, then reduce the heat and cover and simmer for 20 minutes. Puree in a food processor.

 5 portions

Chicken *is a growth food, as it is packed with protein and vitamin B_{12}, which is not found in plant foods. Chicken also naturally contains fat, which is used for energy and growth. It is very important that children aged 6 to 9 months start to regularly eat foods containing adequate amounts of protein.*

SUPERFOODS

Fruity chicken with butternut squash

This is also good made with sweet potato.

1 tablespoon vegetable oil
½ cup chopped onion
5 ounces boneless, skinless chicken breast, cut into chunks
1 medium butternut squash, peeled, seeded, and chopped,
   or 1 medium sweet potato, peeled and chopped
1½ cups unsalted chicken stock
1 small apple, peeled, cored, and chopped

Heat the oil in a saucepan and sauté the onion until softened. Add the chicken breast and sauté for 3 to 4 minutes. Add the butternut squash or sweet potato, pour in the stock, cover, bring to a boil, and simmer for about 10 minutes. Add the apple and cook until the chicken is cooked through and the butternut squash is tender (about 10 minutes). Puree in a food processor to the desired consistency.

 6 portions

Butternut squash
is very appealing to babies, as they love its sweet taste— and it is a very good source of the antioxidant beta-carotene.

SUPERFOODS

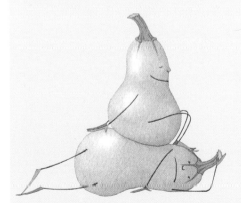

7 to 9 months   59

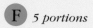

Lamb *provides a good source of B vitamins, zinc, and iron. Babies are born with a store of iron that lasts for about six months, so after this time it is important to ensure that they get the iron they need from their diet.*

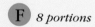 8 portions

Red meat *provides the best and most easily absorbed source of iron. A baby's iron requirements are particularly high between 6 and 12 months.*

Healthy eating:

Never show your own dislike of food to your child—personally I am not madly keen on liver, but my three children loved it as babies!

Sweet potato and lamb casserole

Combining lamb with sweet potato gives it a nice soft texture.

1 lamb rib chop, trimmed of bone and fat and diced

2 scallions, thinly sliced

1 large sweet potato, peeled and chopped

1 medium tomato, peeled, seeded, and chopped

Pinch of dried rosemary or mixed herbs

½ cup unsalted chicken stock or water

Preheat the oven to 350°F. Put all the ingredients into a small casserole dish, cover, and bake in the oven for 10 to 15 minutes or until bubbling. Reduce the heat to 300°F and continue to bake for about 45 minutes or until the lamb is tender. Blend to a puree or chop into small pieces for older babies.

Old-fashioned beef casserole

The onion and carrots in this recipe give the beef a wonderful flavor and the long, slow cooking makes it lovely and tender.

1 medium onion, sliced

1½ tablespoons vegetable oil

8 ounces lean stewing beef (blade or round), cut into chunks

2 medium carrots, peeled and sliced

1 large potato, peeled and diced

1 tablespoon chopped fresh parsley

2 cups unsalted chicken or beef stock

Preheat the oven to 300°F. Sauté the onion in the oil in a flameproof casserole until lightly golden. Add the beef and sauté until browned. Add the carrots, potato, and parsley, pour in the stock, and bring the mixture to a boil.

Cover and transfer the casserole to the oven and bake until the meat is really tender (about 2 hours). Add extra stock if necessary. Blend to a puree of the desired consistency or, for older babies, chop into small pieces.

My first fish puree

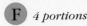

4½ ounces flounder fillet,
   skinned

6 peppercorns

1 bay leaf

Sprig of parsley

½ cup milk

2 medium carrots, peeled and sliced

1¼ cups boiling water

⅓ cup frozen peas

1 tablespoon unsalted butter

1 tablespoon all-purpose flour

¼ cup grated Cheddar cheese

Put the fillet into a saucepan together with the peppercorns, bay leaf, and parsley, and pour in the milk. Simmer until the fish is cooked (about 5 minutes). Strain and reserve the cooking liquid, but discard the peppercorns, bay leaf, and parsley. Flake the fish with a fork, checking to make sure there are no bones.

Put the carrots into a saucepan and pour in the boiling water. Cover and cook over medium heat for 15 minutes, add the peas, and cook for an additional 5 minutes. Drain, reserving the water.

To make the cheese sauce, melt the butter in a saucepan and stir in the flour to make a roux, then gradually whisk in the reserved cooking liquid from the fish. Bring to a boil and simmer until thickened (1 to 2 minutes). Remove from the heat and stir in the grated cheese. Mix in the drained vegetables and the flaked fish. Blend to a smooth puree for young babies and, if necessary, you can add a little more milk or some of the cooking water from the carrots and peas to thin it out.

Fish *is an excellent low-fat source of protein and it is important to encourage a liking for fish early on. I find that one of the best fish to introduce to young babies is flounder, as it purees to a smooth consistency. Here I have mixed it with a creamy cheese sauce and vegetables, so this recipe provides an excellent source of protein, calcium, and vitamins.*

SUPERFOODS

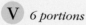
Fillet of salmon with sweet potato

It's important to give oily fish to babies.

1 medium sweet potato, peeled and chopped (1½ cups)
4½ ounces salmon fillet, skinned
⅓ cup freshly squeezed orange juice

½ cup grated Cheddar cheese
Generous pat of unsalted butter
2 tablespoons milk

Put the sweet potato into a steamer and steam for 10 minutes or until tender. You can also cook the potato in a pan with water.

Meanwhile, place the salmon in a suitable dish, pour in the orange juice, and top with the cheese. Microwave on high for about 2 minutes or until the fish flakes easily with a fork. Flake the fish, carefully removing any bones. Mix the sweet potato together with the butter and milk and puree in a blender together with the flaked fish and its sauce. For older babies, mash the sweet potato together with the butter and milk and then mix the flaked fish with the mashed sweet potato.

Vegetable puree with tomato and cheese

Mixing vegetables together with some grated Cheddar cheese and fresh tomatoes gives them a lovely flavor. This puree will provide your baby with both vitamin C and beta-carotene.

2 large carrots, peeled and sliced
1¼ cups chopped cauliflower florets
Generous pat of unsalted butter
2 medium tomatoes, peeled, seeded, and roughly choppcd
¾ cup grated Cheddar cheese

Put the carrots into a saucepan and just cover with boiling water. Cover and cook for 12 minutes, then add the cauliflower and cook for 6 minutes. Meanwhile, melt the butter and sauté the tomatoes for about 2 minutes or until slightly mushy, then stir in the grated cheese until melted. Blend the vegetables together with the cheese and tomato sauce.

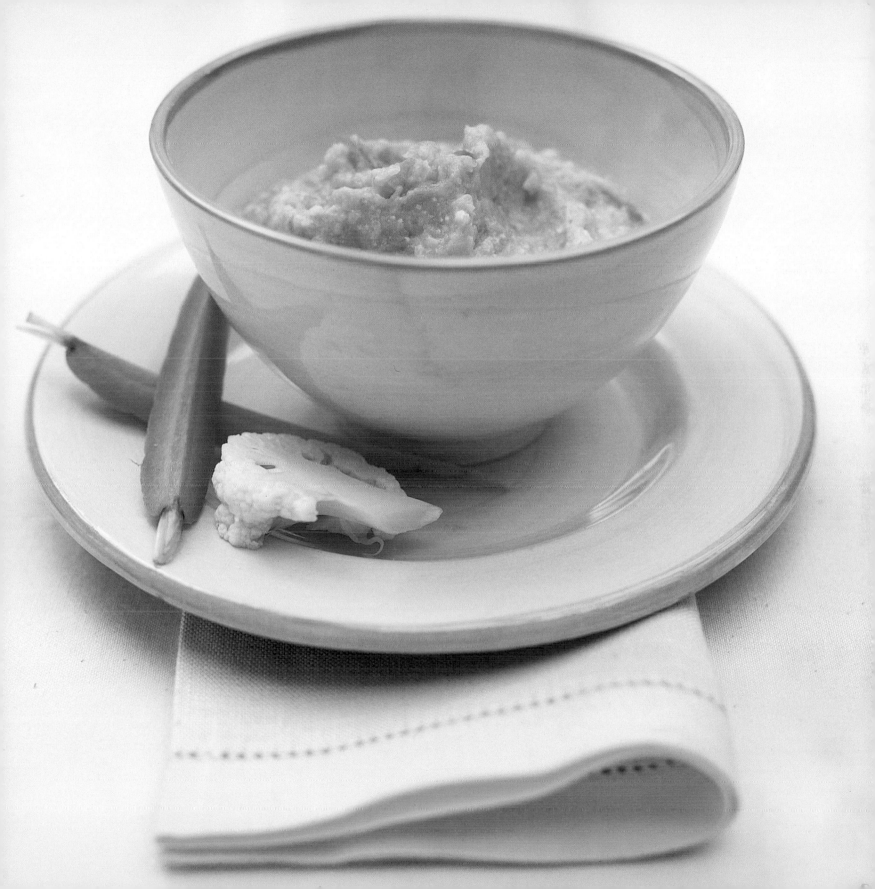

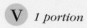 *1 portion*

Bananas and cherries *contain high levels of potassium, which works with sodium to maintain the body's water balance, regulate blood pressure, and maintain a normal heartbeat.*

 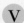 *4 portions*

Tofu *is soybean curd made from soy milk. It is a perfect vegetarian source of protein and rich in many nutrients, including iron, potassium, and calcium. It is a good source of calcium, and eating tofu may help to prevent certain forms of heart disease and cancer.*

  2 portions

Strawberries *contain more vitamin C than other berry fruits. Six strawberries will give an adult almost twice the daily recommended amount. They are also a good source of fiber and beta-carotene and can help protect the body against cancer.*

Cherry and banana puree

6 sweet cherries

1 very small banana

1 teaspoon baby rice cereal (optional)

Wash the cherries, remove the stems, and put the fruit into a small saucepan. Just cover with boiling water, then cover and simmer for about 4 minutes. Allow the cherries to cool down a little, remove the pits, and press through a sieve to get rid of the skins. Mash the banana and mix with the strained cherries. If you like, stir in the baby rice cereal.

Apricot, papaya, and tofu

Although tofu has almost no taste of its own, it combines well with either fruit or vegetables to make a creamy puree. There are two types of tofu—soft or firm.

½ cup chopped dried apricots

1 cup boiling water

1 large papaya, peeled, seeded, and chopped

4 ounces soft tofu

Put the apricots in a small saucepan and pour in the boiling water. Cover and cook until tender (about 5 minutes). Drain the apricots and puree together with the papaya and tofu until smooth.

Strawberry, peach, and apple puree

This is delicious on its own or mixed with a little baby rice cereal or mashed banana.

4 strawberries

1 large juicy peach, peeled, pitted, and cut into pieces

1 apple, peeled, cored, and cut into pieces

Put the fruit in a small, heavy-bottomed saucepan, cover, and simmer for 4 to 5 minutes. Blend to a puree.

Apple, pear, and prune with oats

You could also make this recipe with soft, ready-to-eat dried figs instead of prunes.

2 tablespoons quick-cooking (not instant) oats
¼ cup unsweetened apple juice
1 small apple, peeled, cored, and chopped
2 pitted prunes, chopped
1 small pear, peeled, cored, and chopped

Put the oats, apple juice, and 2 tablespoons water in a saucepan, bring to a boil, and simmer for 2 minutes. Add the chopped apple, prunes, and pear and cover and simmer for 3 minutes, stirring occasionally. Puree to the desired consistency.

My favorite oatmeal

This was my children's favorite breakfast when they were babies. Not only does it taste great, but it is also packed full of nutritious ingredients. Dried apricots are a good source of beta-carotene and iron and also contain fiber.

½ cup milk
¼ cup rolled (not instant) oats
6 dried apricots, chopped
1 large ripe pear, peeled, cored, and cut into pieces

Put the milk, oats, and apricots in a small saucepan, bring to a boil, and then simmer, stirring occasionally, for 3 minutes. Puree together with the chopped pear with a hand blender.

 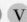 *2 portions*

Prunes *are a good source of instant energy, fiber, and iron. They help with constipation, as they are a natural laxative.*

Healthy eating:

For older children, prunes for breakfast are sometimes a good idea.

  4 portions

Oats *help stabilize blood sugar and help to give long-lasting energy. They are also rich in a form of soluble fiber that protects intestinal surfaces and helps to keep the body's cholesterol levels down.*

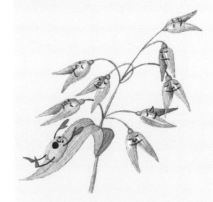

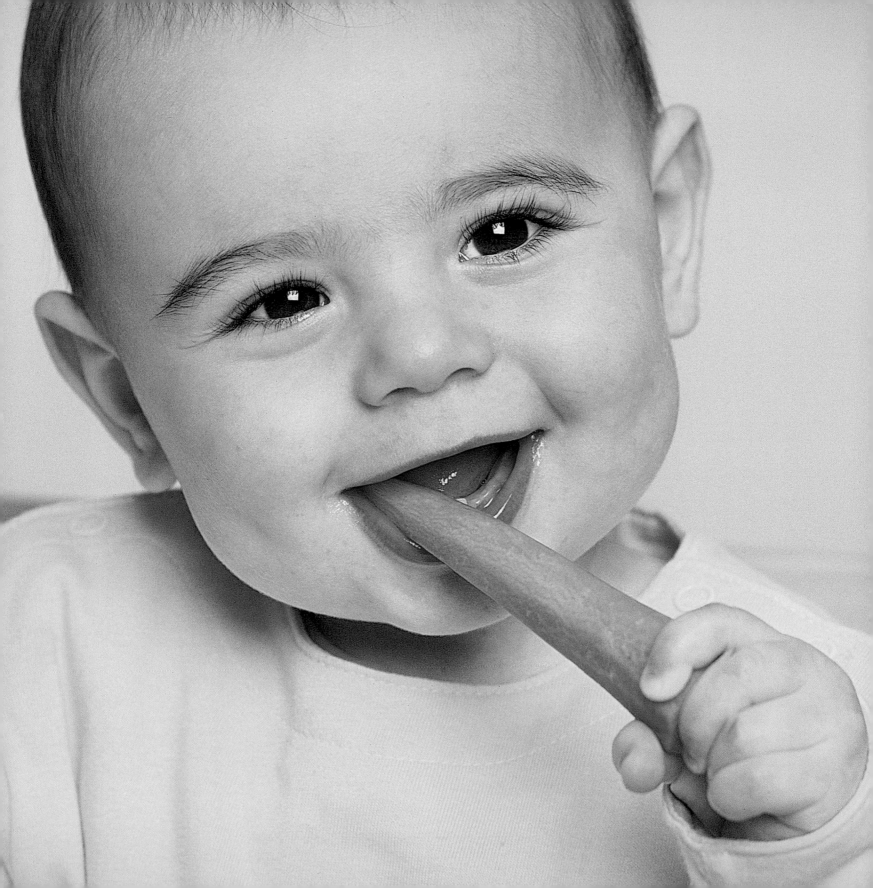

9 to 12 months:
growing independence

Your baby will probably be much more proficient at chewing, and chopped or mashed food can replace purees. Many babies refuse to be spoon-fed, so finger foods become an important part of the diet.

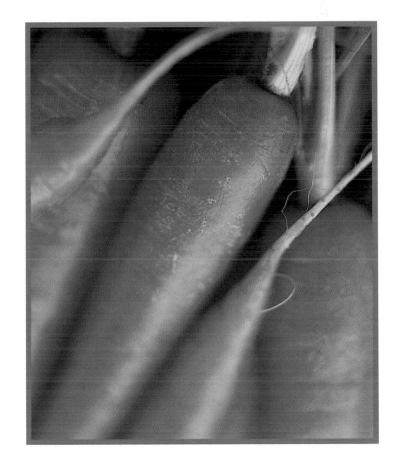

Moving on up

The final quarter of a baby's first year is a time of rapid change, as babies will progress from sitting to crawling and maybe even walking. This is a time of growing independence and your baby will be delighted by this new freedom. During this stage, many babies refuse to be spoon-fed and only want to feed themselves. As your child's hand-eye coordination matures, he will find it much easier to feed himself, and finger foods will become an increasingly important part of your baby's diet.

Encourage your baby to experiment with using a spoon as soon as he is able to hold one. It will be messy at first and he may well end up biting the wrong end, but eventually the food will actually reach its intended destination. The more you allow your baby to experiment, the quicker he will learn to feed himself. It is very important to encourage messy play with food, as this enables learning of self-feeding and quicker development as well.

Learning to chew

By this age, your baby should have gained some teeth and graduated to a high chair, so now it is important to introduce coarser textures in order to encourage your baby to chew. Your baby will gradually be eating more solids so that eventually solid food becomes the main part of the meal. Variety is important, so try introducing lots of different flavors and textures during this stage. Try to give some food mashed, some grated, some diced, and some whole. It is surprising what a few teeth and strong gums can get through.

Milk feedings

Your baby may be drinking less milk as her appetite for solid food increases, but she still needs 17 to 28 ounces of her usual milk per day. Continue with breast milk or formula until your baby is one year old, as cow's milk is too low in iron and vitamin D. Milk is particularly important for calcium, which is necessary for developing strong, healthy bones and teeth. Cow's milk can be used with your baby's cereal or in other forms like cheese sauce or yogurt.

If your baby wants extra drinks, offer cooled boiled water. The sooner your baby can drink from a sippy cup, the better. There are lots of different sippy cups to choose from. A sippy cup with a long spout that is not rigid makes a good transition from a bottle. Aim to dispense with bottles by the age of one year. Most milk feedings are better given in a sippy cup. If it helps to settle your baby, you can keep a breast- or bottle-feeding as a comfort before bedtime.

Which foods to choose

With the exception of raw or lightly cooked eggs, peanuts, whole nuts, shellfish, and unpasteurized cheeses, your baby should now be able to eat most foods. At this age, your baby should be eating three to four servings of starchy food, three to four servings of fruit and vegetables, and at least one serving of meat, chicken, or fish, or two servings of a vegetable protein (soy, peas, beans, lentils, and smooth nut butters), per day.

You can also now give low-sugar whole-grain adult breakfast cereals like oatmeal, granola, and shredded wheat and maybe add chopped fresh or dried fruits and some toasted wheat germ for a nutritious breakfast. Eggs are also a good food for breakfast, but you must make sure that the yolk and white are cooked until solid.

Your baby will probably also be following a more predictable sleeping pattern, which should help to make mealtimes more regular. Whenever possible let your baby sit in his high chair close to the table and enjoy eating with the rest of the family.

Healthy eating: *Drinks at mealtimes should be given after your child has had most of his food to prevent him from filling himself up with liquid.*

Good foods for your baby

• Starchy foods including bread, pasta, rice, cereal, and potato (can be of normal adult texture).

• Lean red meat—this provides the best source of iron.

• Calcium-rich foods like cheese and yogurt—these are important for healthy bones and teeth.

• Eggs—a good source of protein.

• Plenty of fresh fruit and vegetables.

• Remember that babies need more of their diet to come from energy-rich fats and dairy products than adults do, so give them foods like macaroni and cheese, baked potato and cheese, and rice pudding.

• Oily fish contain essential fatty acids that are very healthy. You could make salmon fish cakes with mashed potato, or mashed sardines (don't remove the soft bones, instead mash them in with the fish, as this is a good source of calcium) and use them as a sandwich filling.

• If your child doesn't like eating meat, encourage her to eat other foods that are rich in iron, such as whole-grain cereals and bread, green leafy vegetables, and legumes. Iron in foods of animal origin is much more easily absorbed, but if you include a good source of vitamin C (kiwifruit, orange juice) at the same meal, this will improve the absorption.

Foods to avoid

• Whole nuts.

• Salt or soy sauce.

• Artificial sweeteners.

• Added fiber in the form of bran, which can affect your baby's ability to absorb calcium, zinc, and iron and other vitamins and minerals.

What to do if your baby chokes

If your baby chokes, do not try to fish the food from his mouth, as you may only end up pushing it further down his throat. Tip him face down over your lap with his head lower than his stomach and slap him firmly between the shoulder blades to dislodge the food.

Finger foods

As your baby develops better finger control (this usually happens at around eight months), introducing finger foods will help to develop the all-important skills of biting, chewing, and self-feeding. Finger foods should be big enough for your baby to pick up and easy to hold, and they should not have any seeds, pits, or bones in them. You should also avoid small, hard foods like whole grapes that might cause your baby to choke. Just because your baby has teeth doesn't mean that she knows how to chew food. Instead, young babies are quite likely to bite off a piece of food, try to swallow it whole, and choke on it (see box, above), so never leave a child alone while eating.

To begin with, as your baby learns to feed herself, she will probably drop a lot of her food on the floor. This can all seem very charming and amusing to begin with, but it can become a tragic waste of food. To prevent this happening, it's a good idea to invest in a plastic splash mat that can be laid under her high chair so that the food falls on a clean surface and can then be recycled. It will also ease the chore of clearing up behind her after every meal.

Tip: *Finger foods are great for occupying your child while you prepare his meal.*

Ideas for first finger foods

Offering a selection of these to your baby will get him used to chewing many different textures.

• Sticks of vegetables like carrots or parsnip make good finger food. But raw vegetables can be difficult to chew, so it is much better to lightly steam vegetables or cook them in a little boiling water for a few minutes so that they are still crunchy but not quite so hard. When your baby seems to cope well with these, try introducing cucumber, and as your baby gains more teeth, introduce raw vegetables like carrots.

• Fruits make good finger food, and if your baby finds it difficult to chew, to begin with give soft fruits that melt in the mouth, like banana, peach, and kiwifruit.

• Dried fruits like apricot or apple make good nutritious finger foods.

• Many babies who are teething really enjoy biting into something cold, as it soothes the gums. A banana put into the freezer for a couple of hours makes an excellent teething aid (freeze the banana with the skin on), as does a chilled cucumber stick.

• Fingers of toast tend to work better than plain bread, as they do not fall to pieces so readily.

• For fun finger food you can cut sandwiches, cheese, or large vegetables into shapes using cookie cutters. Good sandwich fillings are mashed banana, cream cheese, egg salad, peanut butter, tuna salad, and hummus.

• Cooked pasta shapes.

• Rice cakes.

• Sticks of mild cheese.

• Fish sticks.

• Slices or small chunks of chicken or turkey and miniature meatballs made of ground chicken, turkey, lamb, or beef.

Equipment

This is a good time to invest in suction-based bowls and spill-proof cups. A splash mat (plastic sheet) under your child's chair will enable finger foods to be recycled. It can be a good idea to have two bowls of food, one for your baby to play with (preferably with a suction pad) and one from which you spoon feed your baby. You can expect a mess, but you want to do your best to stop your child from tipping his food onto the floor. A large wipe-clean bib will help to protect your baby's clothes.

Tip: *Don't expect your child to have good table manners at this age. Exploring the feel of his food is all part of the learning process. The more you allow your child to experiment, the quicker he will get the hang of feeding himself.*

Meal planner

Other ideas for desserts are fresh fruit like a banana or grated apple, fruit puree, and occasionally ice cream, rice pudding, or fruit yogurt.

	BREAKFAST	MID-MORNING	LUNCH	MID-AFTERNOON	SUPPER	BEDTIME
DAY 1	Scrambled egg and toast Yogurt	Breast or formula milk	Baby's Bolognese (page 85) Fruit	Breast or formula milk	Mashed Potato and Carrot with Broccoli and Swiss Cheese (page 74) Fruit	Breast or formula milk
DAY 2	My Favorite Oatmeal (page 65) Fruit	Breast or formula milk	Finger-Picking Chicken Balls (page 84) Yogurt	Breast or formula milk	Tasty Egg and Tomato with Cheese Sauce (page 78) Fresh Peach Melba (page 85)	Breast or formula milk
DAY 3	Cereal Fruit	Breast or formula milk	Cherub's Couscous (page 78) Strawberry Rice Pudding (page 86)	Breast or formula milk	Broccoli in Cheese Sauce (page 75) Fruit	Breast or formula milk
DAY 4	French Toast (page 86) Fruit	Breast or formula milk	Mini Shepherd's Pie (page 83) First Fruit Puree (page 40)	Breast or formula milk	Pasta Risotto (page 80) Strawberry, Peach, and Apple Puree (page 64)	Breast or formula milk
DAY 5	Cereal Apple, Apricot, and Pear Puree (page 46)	Breast or formula milk	Fillet of Salmon with Sweet Potato (page 62) Fruit	Breast or formula milk	Fun Finger Foods with Dips (page 77) Strawberry Rice Pudding (page 86)	Breast or formula milk
DAY 6	Scrambled egg and toast Yogurt	Breast or formula milk	Carrot, Cheese, and Tomato Risotto (page 74) Fresh Peach Melba (page 85)	Breast or formula milk	Tender Casserole of Lamb (page 84) Fruit	Breast or formula milk
DAY 7	Toast with peanut butter Fruit	Breast or formula milk	Finger-Picking Chicken Balls (page 84) Fruit	Breast or formula milk	Cheesy Mushroom and Tomato Sauce with Pasta Stars (page 75) Yogurt	Breast or formula milk

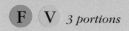

SUPERFOODS

Swiss cheese *has a slightly sweet taste that appeals to babies. Cheese is a good source of concentrated calories, protein, and calcium.*

Healthy eating:
Stronger-tasting vegetables like spinach are good combined with potato.

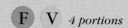

SUPERFOODS

Spinach *is rich in chlorophyll, the green pigment found in plants that helps prevent and treat anemia. Spinach is a good source of beta-carotene and vitamin C, so do not overcook it or you will destroy a lot of its content. But despite popular opinion—and Popeye—it is not a particularly good source of iron.*

Tiny pasta with Swiss cheese, spinach, and corn

Spinach has quite a strong taste on its own but blends well with a cheese sauce, and the corn adds a slightly sweet taste that babies like. You can choose any tiny pasta shape, but I particularly like orzo, which is a pasta that looks like grains of rice.

3 tablespoons orzo or other small pasta shape
1 tablespoon unsalted butter
1 tablespoon all-purpose flour
½ cup your baby's usual milk
½ cup grated Swiss cheese

2 cups fresh spinach, tough stems removed, or ¼ cup thawed frozen spinach
⅔ cup cooked frozen corn

Cook the pasta according to the instructions on the package. Melt the butter, stir in the flour, and cook for 30 seconds. Gradually whisk in the milk to make a smooth white sauce. Bring to a boil and simmer for 1 to 2 minutes. Remove from the heat and stir in the cheese until melted. If using fresh spinach, carefully wash it and put in a saucepan, sprinkle with a little water, and cook until tender (about 3 minutes). Squeeze out all the water. Combine the spinach (fresh or frozen) with the cheese sauce and puree in a food mill. Stir the cooked pasta and corn into the spinach and cheese sauce.

Spinach with mushrooms and potato

½ small onion, chopped
1 tablespoon vegetable oil
1½ cups diced button mushrooms
1 large potato, peeled and diced
½ cup unsalted vegetable stock
2 cups fresh spinach, tough stems removed, or ⅓ cup thawed frozen spinach

Sauté the onion in the oil until softened. Add the mushrooms and sauté for 2 to 3 minutes. Add the potato and pour in the vegetable stock. Bring to a boil, then cover and simmer for 10 minutes. Add the spinach (carefully washed if fresh) and cook for 2 to 3 minutes. Mash with a fork or puree in a food processor.

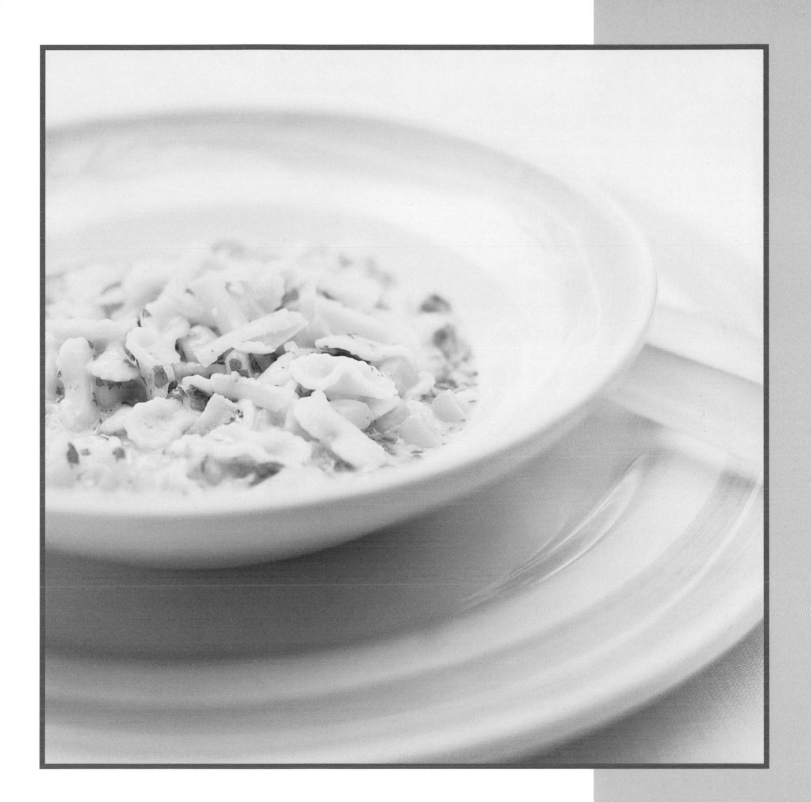

F **V** *4 portions*

Broccoli *is king of the healthy vegetable superstars. Its phytochemicals have important properties, especially against cancer. It provides an excellent source of vitamin C and beta-carotene. The darker the florets, the higher the amount of antioxidants. Broccoli should be steamed, as boiling almost halves its vitamin C content.*

 F **V** *4 portions*

Carrots *are more nutritious when cooked, unlike many other vegetables. Cooking breaks open the plant cells so antioxidants and other plant chemicals can be absorbed much better. Carrots contain large amounts of carotene, an antioxidant that gives carrots their orange color.*

Mashed potato and carrot with broccoli and Swiss cheese

Mashing rather than pureeing your baby's food is a good way to gradually introduce more texture. Combining broccoli with creamy mashed potato and cheese is a great way to encourage babies to eat more greens.

1 medium potato, peeled and diced
1 medium carrot, peeled and sliced
3 or 4 broccoli florets

¼ cup your baby's usual milk
1 pat unsalted butter
⅓ cup grated Swiss cheese

Put the potato and carrot into a saucepan, cover with boiling water, and cook until tender (about 20 minutes). Meanwhile, steam the broccoli until tender (about 8 minutes). Drain the potato and carrot and mash together with the broccoli, milk, butter, and cheese.

Carrot, cheese, and tomato risotto

This is a very easy to prepare and nutritious rice dish. Babies and toddlers tend to like rice and carrot, and here I have flavored them with sautéed tomatoes and melted cheese for a very tasty meal. Cooked rice is quite soft so is a good way of introducing texture to your baby's food.

¼ cup chopped onion
1 tablespoon unsalted butter
¼ cup long-grain rice
1 large carrot, peeled and sliced
1¼ cups boiling water

3 tomatoes, peeled, seeded, and
chopped
½ cup grated Cheddar cheese

Sauté the onion in half the butter until softened. Stir in the rice until well coated, then add the carrot. Pour in the boiling water, bring back to a boil, then cover and simmer until the rice is cooked and the carrot is tender (15 to 20 minutes). If necessary, add extra water. Meanwhile, melt the remaining butter in a small pan, add the tomatoes, and sauté until mushy (2 to 3 minutes). Stir in the cheese until melted. The water from the rice should have been absorbed but if not, drain off any excess. Stir the tomato and cheese mixture into the cooked rice.

Cheesy mushroom and tomato sauce with pasta stars

 F V *3 portions*

The addition of tiny pasta shapes to this tasty tomato sauce enriched with mushrooms and cheese is a gentle way to introduce a little texture to your baby's food.

2 tablespoons tiny pasta stars (or shapes)
2 tablespoons unsalted butter
½ small clove garlic
1½ cups sliced button mushrooms

3 tomatoes, peeled, seeded, and
  roughly chopped
¼ cup grated Cheddar cheese

Cook the pasta according to the instructions on the package. Melt the butter in a saucepan and sauté the garlic for about 30 seconds. Add the sliced mushrooms and sauté for 3 minutes. Add the tomatoes and cook, covered, until mushy (3 to 4 minutes). Stir in the cheese until melted. Puree the vegetable and cheese mixture, then stir in the cooked pasta.

Broccoli in cheese sauce

 F V *3 portions*

For older babies this also makes a good pasta sauce. Simply increase the amount of milk to 1¼ cups and add an extra 3 tablespoons of Swiss cheese to the sauce and then mix with cooked small pasta shapes. You could also make this with cauliflower.

1 cup small broccoli florets
1 tablespoon unsalted butter
1 tablespoon all-purpose flour
1 cup your baby's usual milk

Pinch of grated nutmeg
¼ cup grated Cheddar cheese
¼ cup grated Swiss cheese

Steam the broccoli florets until tender (about 8 minutes). Alternatively, put in a saucepan, cover with boiling water, and cook until tender. Meanwhile, to prepare the cheese sauce, melt the butter in a saucepan and stir in the flour to make a roux. Gradually whisk in the milk and the nutmeg to make a smooth white sauce. Bring to a boil and then simmer for 2 minutes. Remove from the heat and stir in the cheeses until melted. Chop the broccoli into small pieces and mix with the cheese sauce. Alternatively, puree the broccoli and cheese sauce.

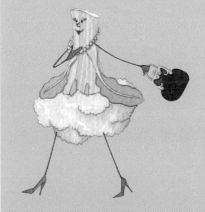
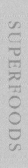

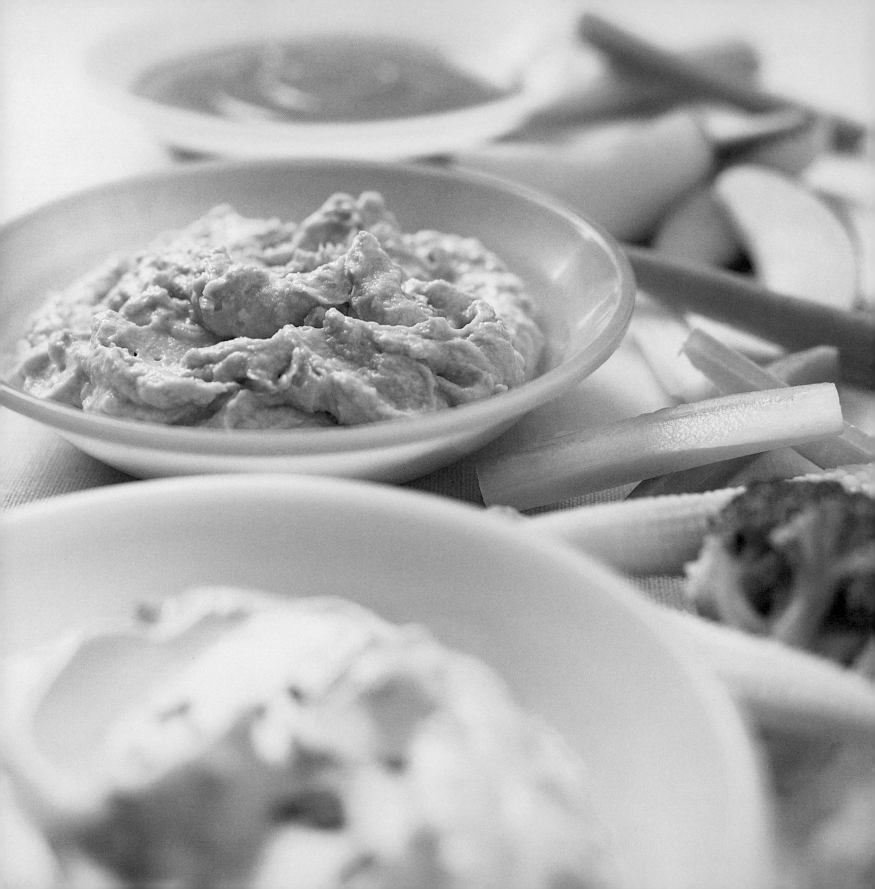

Fun finger foods with dips

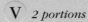 *2 portions*

Once your baby is able to hold food, finger foods that allow her to feed herself will become an increasingly important part of her diet. Fresh fruit and vegetables served with tasty dips make an appealing and nutritious meal. Here are three of my favorites, each of which is particularly high up on the SuperFood scale.

Creamy avocado dip

½ avocado, mashed

2 tablespoons cream cheese

1 tomato, peeled, seeded, and chopped

1 teaspoon snipped chives (optional)

Mash the avocado together with the cream cheese and stir in the chopped tomato and chives, if using.

Serve with vegetables like carrot, cucumber, bell pepper, and celery. Give steamed vegetables to young babies and when they are better able to chew and swallow, move on to raw vegetables.

Cream cheese, tomato, and chive dip

2 ounces cream cheese

3 tablespoons sour cream or crème fraîche

1 teaspoon ketchup

1 tomato, peeled, seeded, and chopped

1½ teaspoons snipped chives

Mix together the cream cheese, sour cream, and ketchup and stir in the chopped tomato and chives.

Raspberry yogurt dip

½ cup fresh or frozen raspberries

2 tablespoons superfine sugar

1 cup plain yogurt, drained in a coffee filter overnight to thicken

Puree the raspberries, press through a sieve, and stir in the sugar. Stir the raspberry puree into the strained yogurt. Serve with fruits like strawberries, pear, apple, and peach.

SUPERFOODS

Avocados *are sometimes thought of as a vegetable but they are actually a fruit and contain more nutrients than any other fruit. Avocados have the highest protein content of any fruit and are rich in monounsaturated fat, the "good" type of fat, which helps prevent heart disease. The high calorie content of avocados makes them a good food for growing children.*

Tomatoes *are rich in lycopene (see page 75) and potassium, which is important for healthy blood and helps counteract the negative effects of salt. One of the factors of the good health of the Mediterranean people may be that their diet is rich in fruit and vegetables, including tomatoes.*

Raspberries *are rich in vitamin C, which is needed for growth, healthy skin, bones, and teeth and also helps the body to absorb iron from food. Raspberries are higher in folic acid and zinc than most fruits.*

Eggs *are packed with goodness. Remember, they contain all the nutrients needed to support a chick. Eggs provide an excellent source of protein, zinc, and vitamins A, D, E, and B$_{12}$. Don't worry about their high cholesterol—in the long run, it has very little effect compared to things like obesity and smoking.*

Tasty egg and tomato with cheese sauce

Eggs provide us with protein, vitamins, and minerals, and egg yolk is a good source of iron, which is important for a baby's brain development. Raw or lightly cooked eggs should not be given to babies or young children because of the risk of salmonella. It's fine to give eggs after six months, provided the white and yolk are cooked until solid.

1 egg
1 pat unsalted butter
1 tomato, peeled, seeded, and roughly chopped
2 tablespoons grated Cheddar cheese

Put the egg into a small saucepan, cover with water, and bring to a boil. Boil until the white and yolk are solid (about 10 minutes). Melt the butter in a small saucepan. Stir in the chopped tomato and cook until mushy (about 2 minutes). Remove from the heat and stir in the grated cheese until melted. Remove the shell from the egg and mash the white and yolk with a fork. Mix with the tomato and cheese.

Couscous *is made from semolina wheat and is popular in Middle Eastern cuisine. You can find it in most supermarkets next to the rice section. It's fairly high in minerals and vitamins, and has a mild taste and wonderful soft texture. It is also very quick and easy to prepare.*

Cherub's couscous

1 cup unsalted chicken stock
½ cup couscous
1 tablespoon unsalted butter
¼ cup chopped onion
½ cup diced zucchini
2 tomatoes, peeled, seeded, and chopped
½ cup diced cooked chicken

Bring the chicken stock to a boil and pour over the couscous, stir with a fork, and set aside for 6 minutes, by which time it will have absorbed the stock. Meanwhile, melt the butter in a saucepan and sauté the onion for 2 minutes. Add the zucchini and sauté for about 4 minutes, then add the tomatoes and cook for 1 minute. Fluff the couscous with a fork and mix in the zucchini and tomato mixture together with the chicken.

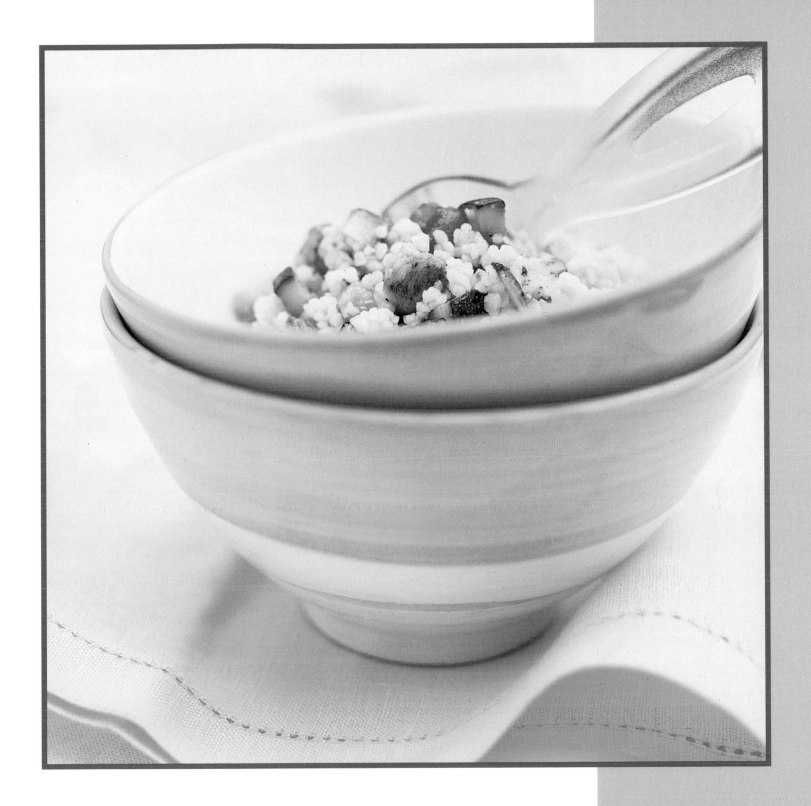

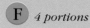 *4 portions*

Cow's milk *is a nutritious ingredient in food for infants aged 9 to 12 months, as it is naturally high in protein, fat, and calcium and contains many other vitamins and minerals. Remember, however, that cow's milk should not be given as a drink before one year of age, as it is low in iron and too high in protein.*

Chopped chicken with diced vegetables in cheese sauce

Combining finely chopped food with a creamy cheese sauce makes lumpier textures easier to swallow. If you don't have any cooked chicken, you could poach 2 ounces of raw chicken in stock for about 10 minutes. You could also use flaked fish instead of the cooked chicken.

½ cup small broccoli florets	1 cup your baby's usual milk
½ cup sliced carrot	⅓ cup grated Edam or Cheddar cheese
2 tablespoons unsalted butter	2 ounces cooked chicken, diced
2 tablespoons all-purpose flour	

Steam the broccoli and carrot until tender. Cut the broccoli into small pieces and dice the carrot. To prepare the cheese sauce, melt the butter in a saucepan, stir in the flour, and cook for 1 minute. Gradually whisk in the milk, bring to a boil, and cook until the sauce has thickened. Remove from the heat and stir in the cheese until melted. Mix the chicken and vegetables into the cheese sauce. For young babies, puree to the desired consistency in a blender.

 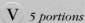 *5 portions*

Pasta *is a great energy food, packed full of carbohydrates, which are broken down to supply all the cells in our bodies with fuel. Sixty percent of the adult diet should be carbohydrates, and introducing starchy-type foods early on is a good idea.*

Pasta risotto

You can vary the vegetables in this tasty and simple to prepare recipe. Try also peas, corn, or diced tomatoes.

½ cup orzo or other small pasta shape	½ cup diced broccoli florets
½ cup diced carrot	2 tablespoons unsalted butter
½ cup diced zucchini	¼ cup grated Cheddar cheese

Put the pasta in a saucepan together with the carrot, cover generously with boiling water, and cook for 5 minutes. Add the zucchini and broccoli and continue to cook for about 7 minutes. Melt the butter in a saucepan, stir in the drained pasta and vegetables, and toss with the Cheddar cheese until the cheese has melted.

SUPERFOODS

Orzo with creamy mushroom and cheese sauce

¾ cup orzo or other small pasta shape

¼ cup chopped onion

2 tablespoons diced red bell pepper

1 tablespoon olive oil

1½ cups diced button mushrooms

1 tablespoon unsalted butter

1 tablespoon all-purpose flour

¾ cup your baby's usual milk

2 tablespoons grated Parmesan cheese

Cook the orzo in boiling water according to the package instructions and drain. Meanwhile, sauté the onion and red pepper in the olive oil until softened (about 5 minutes). Add the mushrooms and sauté for 2 to 3 minutes.

To make the cheese sauce, melt the butter in a small saucepan and stir in the flour to make a roux. Gradually whisk in the milk over medium heat until the sauce has thickened, and finally stir in the cheese. To serve, mix together the orzo, vegetables, and cheese sauce.

Risotto with butternut squash

Cooked rice with vegetables is nice and soft, so it's a good way to introduce texture to your baby's food. Butternut squash is rich in vitamin A. You could also make this with pumpkin instead of squash.

½ cup chopped onion

2 tablespoons unsalted butter

½ cup basmati rice

2 cups boiling water

1 small butternut squash, peeled and chopped

3 tomatoes, peeled, seeded, and chopped

½ cup grated Cheddar cheese

Sauté the onion in half the butter until softened. Stir in the rice until well coated. Pour in the boiling water, cover, and cook for 8 minutes over high heat. Stir in the chopped squash, reduce the heat, and cook, covered, for about 12 minutes or until the water has been absorbed.

Meanwhile, melt the remaining butter in a small pan, add the tomatoes, and sauté for 2 to 3 minutes. Stir in the cheese until melted. Combine the rice with the tomato and cheese sauce.

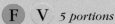 5 portions

Cheese *is a perfect food for children. It provides an excellent source of protein and calcium, important for strong bones and good teeth.*

Healthy eating:
For older children you could serve this dish with some freshly grated Parmesan cheese sprinkled on top.

F   4 portions

Butternut squash *is rich in beta-carotene, the plant form of vitamin A, which helps protect against cancer and boosts your child's immune system.*

SUPERFOODS

SUPERFOODS

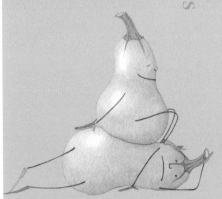

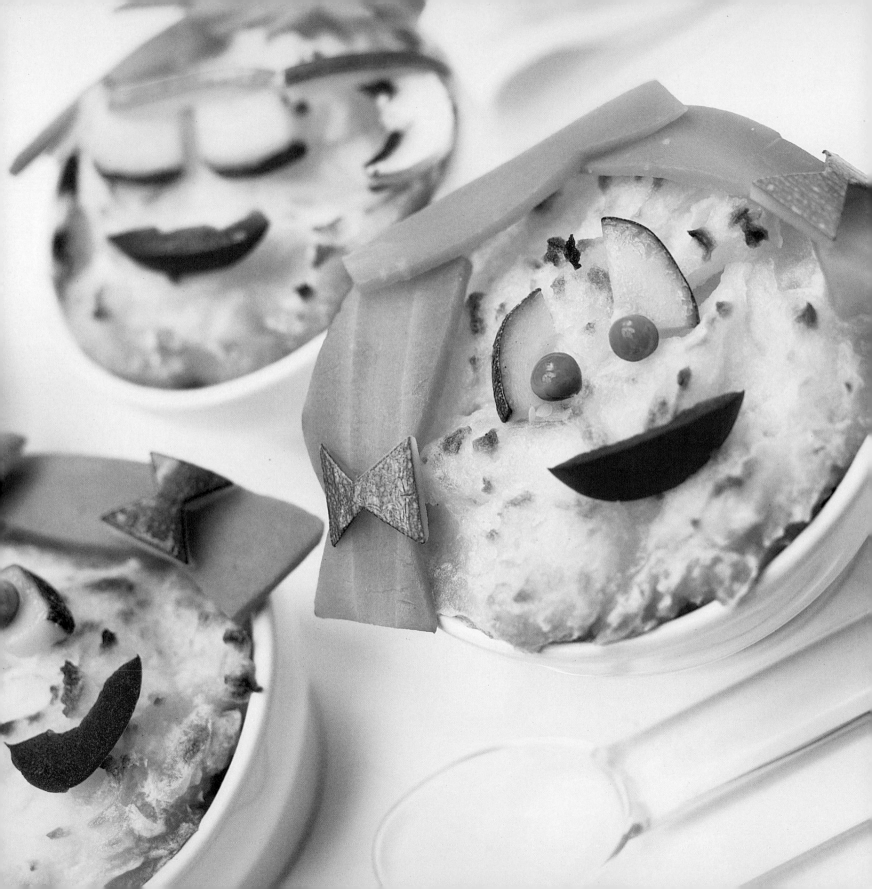

Mini shepherd's pie

Combining ground meat with creamy mashed potatoes gives it a much smoother texture that is easier to swallow. Mashed potatoes and carrots or mashed potatoes and rutabaga make a tasty combination and combine well with ground meat. For babies under 9 months it would be best to puree the cooked ground meat before combining it with the mashed potato.

2 medium potatoes, peeled and diced

2 medium carrots, peeled and sliced

1 tablespoon vegetable oil

1 small clove garlic, minced

¼ cup chopped onion

4 ounces lean ground beef or lamb

1 tomato, peeled, seeded, and chopped

1 teaspoon ketchup

½ cup unsalted chicken stock

1 tablespoon unsalted butter

2 tablespoons your baby's usual milk

Put the potatoes and carrots into a saucepan, pour in boiling water, and cook the vegetables until tender (about 20 minutes). Meanwhile, heat the oil in a small saucepan and sauté the garlic and onion until softened. Add the ground meat and sauté, stirring occasionally, until browned all over. Add the tomato and ketchup and pour in the stock. Cover, bring to a boil, and then simmer for about 20 minutes. When the potatoes and carrots are cooked, drain and return to the saucepan together with the butter and milk, and mash with a potato masher until smooth; you can also put the mixture through a potato ricer. Mix the meat with the mashed potato and carrot.

For young babies, puree the meat in a food processor before mixing it with the mashed potato and carrot. As your baby gets a little older, make this into a mini shepherd's pie and decorate with a face made from vegetables.

Red meat *provides a rich source of iron, and by including it with foods like dark green leafy vegetables or whole-grain bread, you will improve the absorption of the vegetable sources of iron in the meal by three times.*

SUPERFOODS

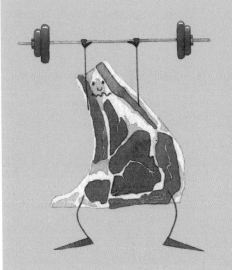

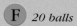

Chicken *is high in
protein, low in fat, and low
in cholesterol. Our bodies
require a certain amount
of protein each day and the
body does not store protein,
so we need to replenish it
each day. Protein provides
the building blocks of all
cells.*

Finger-picking chicken balls

These tasty chicken balls make great finger food.

1 tablespoon light olive oil

1 medium onion, finely chopped

½ cup grated carrot

1 large Granny Smith apple,
   peeled and grated

Two 6-ounce boneless, skinless
   chicken breasts, cut into chunks

1 tablespoon chopped fresh parsley

1 teaspoon chopped fresh thyme or
   ½ teaspoon dried (optional)

½ cup fresh white bread crumbs

1 chicken bouillon cube, crumbled

Salt and freshly ground black pepper

All-purpose flour for coating

Vegetable oil for frying

Heat the olive oil in a pan and sauté half the onion and the grated carrot for 3 minutes,
stirring occasionally. Using your hands, squeeze out a little excess liquid from the grated
apple. Mix together the grated apple, chicken, and sautéed onion and carrot along with the
raw chopped onion, parsley, thyme (if using), bread crumbs, and stock cube and chop for a
few seconds in a food processor. Season with a little salt and pepper.

With your hands, form the mixture into about 20 balls, roll them in flour, and fry in a
little oil until lightly golden and cooked through (4 to 5 minutes).

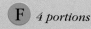

Lamb *is high in protein,
essential for growth, and a
good source of iron, zinc,
and B vitamins. Lamb tends
to be more fatty than beef, so
trim off any excess fat.*

Tender casserole of lamb

Cooking lamb in a casserole with vegetables such as carrots, potatoes, and tomatoes and
broth makes it tender and moist for your baby.

Two 3-ounce lamb rib chops,
   trimmed of fat and bone

½ small onion, chopped

1 large potato, peeled and diced

½ cup diced sweet potato

1 large carrot, peeled and sliced

2 tomatoes, peeled, seeded, and chopped

½ cup unsalted chicken stock

Preheat the oven to 350°F. Put the lamb, vegetables, and stock into a small casserole,
cover, and cook until the lamb is tender (about 1 hour). Chop into small pieces or puree
for young babies.

Baby's Bolognese

Often it is not the taste of red meat that babies dislike but the texture, so here I blend the Bolognese sauce so that the ground meat becomes very easy to chew, and then mix it with soft pasta.

¼ cup finely chopped onion

2 tablespoons finely chopped celery

1 tablespoon vegetable oil

2 tablespoons finely grated carrot

5 ounces lean ground beef

1 tablespoon ketchup

2 tomatoes, peeled, seeded, and chopped

¼ cup unsalted chicken stock

2 ounces spaghetti

Sauté the onion and celery in the vegetable oil for 3 to 4 minutes. Add the grated carrot and cook for 2 minutes. Add the ground beef and stir until browned. Stir in the ketchup, tomatoes, and stock. Bring the mixture to a boil, then reduce the heat, cover, and cook until the meat is cooked through (10 to 15 minutes). Meanwhile, cook the spaghetti according to package instructions until quite soft. Drain and chop into short lengths. Transfer the Bolognese sauce to a food processor and puree to a fairly smooth texture before combining with the pasta.

Fresh peach melba

2 portions

This raspberry sauce is also good served with fresh strawberries.

½ cup fresh or thawed frozen raspberries

1 tablespoon superfine sugar

2 scoops vanilla ice cream

2 peaches, peeled, pitted, and sliced

Make the melba sauce by pureeing the raspberries in a food processor, then push them through a sieve to get rid of the seeds and stir in the sugar until dissolved. Put the ice cream into a dish together with the peach slices and pour the sauce over the top.

Milk *provides an excellent source of protein for growth and calcium, which is important for healthy bones and teeth.*

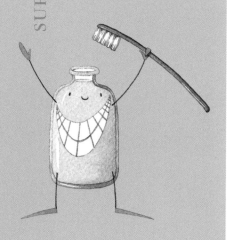

1 to 2 portions

Breads *are now available in a staggering variety. Choose bread made from whole grains. These breads contain all the goodness of the complete wheat husk and wheat germ, and are higher in fiber and a good source of B vitamins. White breads have had a lot of goodness leached from them in the processing.*

Strawberry rice pudding

The secret of a good rice pudding is long, slow cooking. You could leave out the strawberry jam and add some cooked fruit like stewed plums or add some chopped dried fruit instead, like mango or apricots, which can be cooked together with the rice.

¼ cup long-grain rice (not converted)
2 cups your baby's usual milk
¼ teaspoon pure vanilla extract
1½ tablespoons superfine sugar
1 pat unsalted butter
Strawberry jam

Preheat the oven to 300°F. Place the rice, milk, vanilla, and sugar in a greased ovenproof dish and stir well. Dot the surface with the butter. Bake for 30 minutes, then stir. Continue to bake until the rice is tender (1 to 1½ hours). Remove from the oven and serve each portion topped with strawberry jam.

French toast

1 or 2 slices white bread, raisin bread, or French bread
1 egg
2 tablespoons whole milk
1 tablespoon unsalted butter and a little vegetable oil
Sugar and/or ground cinnamon (optional)

Remove the crusts and cut the bread into four triangles or into fingers. Beat together the egg and milk and soak the bread in this mixture for a few seconds. Drain on paper towels. Heat the butter and oil in a frying pan and fry the bread until brown on both sides.

For a sweet version, add a little sugar and/or a pinch of ground cinnamon to the egg mixture and sprinkle a little sugar on the toast after frying.

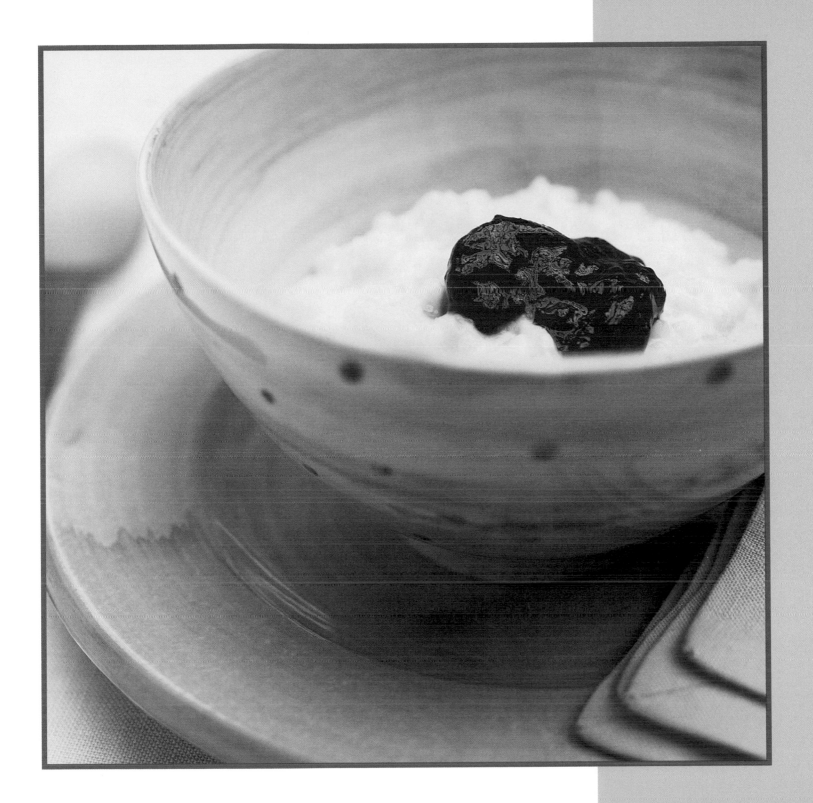

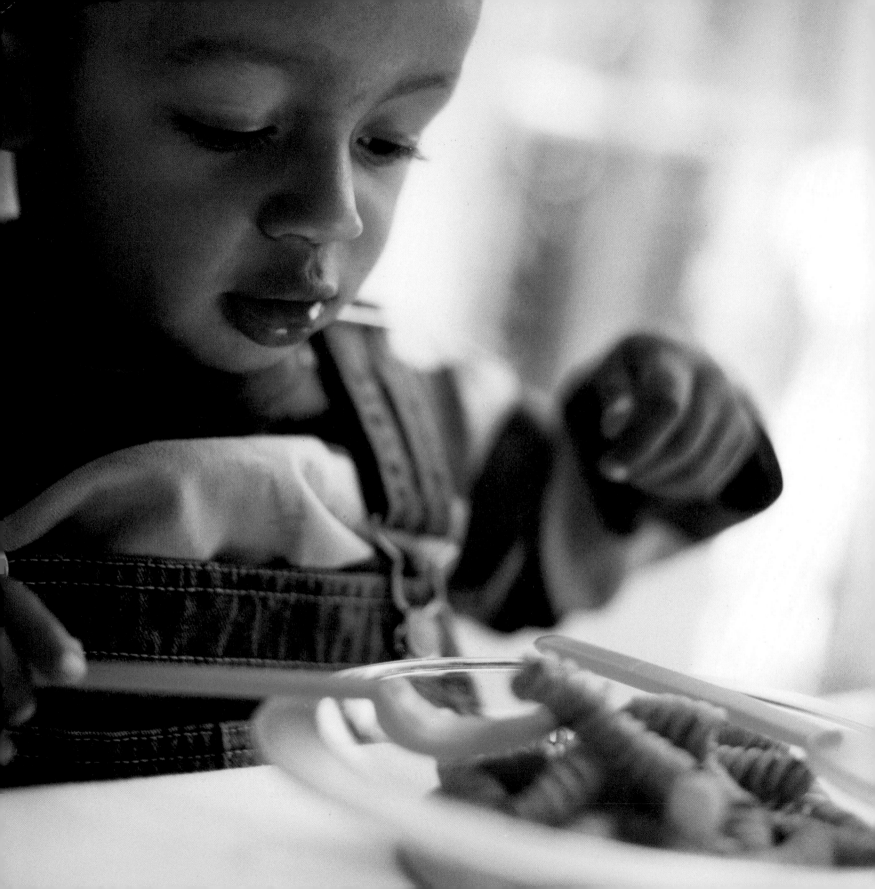

1 to 2 years:
time to explore

From the age of one, solid food will replace much of the milk in your baby's diet. Try introducing a wider variety of foods, presented in an appealing way, and encourage your baby to feed himself.

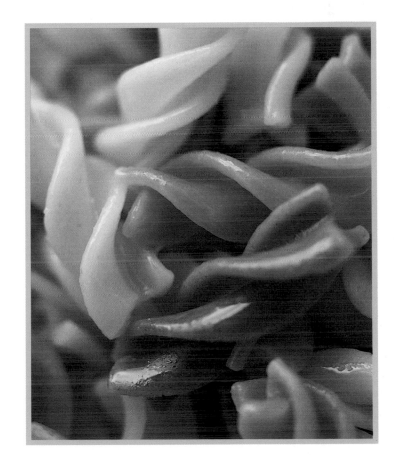

Breakfast power

There is a lot of truth in that old saying "Breakfast like a king, lunch like a knave, and dine like a pauper." However, up to 17 percent of schoolchildren skip breakfast before school. The first meal of the day is the most important, as your child will probably have fasted for up to twelve hours. Our bodies release glucose from our stores shortly before we wake up to help us arise from bed. Once we're awake, the glucose needs to be replaced by food in order to give our brains a kick start. Improving blood sugar by eating a good breakfast after the night's fast raises blood glucose ("fuel for the brain") and will help to improve your child's performance. Recent research has shown that children who eat a nutritionally balanced breakfast worked faster, made significantly fewer mistakes on tasks requiring sustained attention, demonstrated greater physical endurance, and appeared less tired to teachers. Studies have also shown that children who go to school on a good breakfast not only will concentrate better but will also be better able to remember what they are taught.

No one really needs scientists to tell them that it is easier to focus on a mental task if their tummy is not rumbling with hunger. Breakfast sets the pattern for healthy eating during the day and if your child misses breakfast, he will end up craving sweet foods later in the morning because his body will need glucose fast. Breakfast is the ideal time to make sure that your child gets some healthy energy-giving food into his diet, as, unlike with school lunches, you are in control of what your child eats. My favorite ways of serving delicious breakfasts are given here.

Breakfasts for energy and brain power

Children have high energy and nutrient requirements because they are active and growing rapidly, so it is important that their diet is not too high in fiber or low in fat, otherwise your child may feel full before his requirements are met. Choose whole milk and whole milk dairy products and don't give too many high-fiber cereals.

For toddlers, especially, it is important to remember that little people have small stomachs that get full quickly. The food they eat needs to be packed full of as many nutrients as possible. Peanut butter on toast, yogurt, or some cheese and a glass of fruit juice would provide an excellent breakfast for a toddler. Eggs are good for breakfast and very versatile.

While children are still growing, it is important that they get a good supply of vital nutrients like calcium and iron. Children who eat a good breakfast are much less likely to suffer nutritional deficiencies. After all, a simple bowl of cereal with milk will supply both iron and calcium.

For maximum energy and brain power to last throughout the morning a good breakfast should ideally include something from each of these groups:

- Complex carbohydrates: cereal and bread.
- Protein: dairy products, eggs, and nuts.
- Vitamins and minerals: fruit (occasionally vegetables, as in an omelet).

Calcium

Try to include at least one calcium-rich food each day for breakfast (see the meal planner on page 93). A good supply of calcium is essential to ensure the development of strong, healthy bones and this is particularly important during childhood and the teenage years when there is rapid growth. Calcium is also essential for the development of teeth, being a key part of the tooth structure. Milk and dairy products are the main source of calcium in our diet. (See also page 14.)

Eggs

Eggs are rich in essential nutrients and almost all the nutrients are concentrated in the yolk, which contains protein, fat, vitamins, minerals, and folic acid. Eggs are a good source of iron.

Very young children should not eat lightly cooked or raw eggs because of the risk of salmonella. Very fresh eggs contain fewer bacteria than older eggs, so check the "sell by" date on the carton and buy the freshest eggs you can.

The importance of iron

Iron deficiency is the commonest nutritional deficiency in young children. Recent surveys have shown that one in every five babies aged ten to twelve months has a daily intake of iron below the recommended level. Two of the main symptoms are tiredness and lack of concentration. Fortified cereals and whole-wheat bread are good sources of iron. But to improve the absorption of the iron you will need to include vitamin C–rich fruit like kiwi or berry fruits or vitamin C–rich juice like orange juice or cranberry juice. (See also page 16.)

Bread and cereals

A bowl of cereal can make a healthy start to the day, but you will need to choose carefully. Many of the attractively packaged breakfast cereals designed specifically for children are highly refined and have lost most of their valuable nutrients. Don't be misled by claims that they are fortified with important vitamins and minerals, since many more nutrients are taken out than put back. These cereals also tend to be very high in sugar (sometimes nearly 50 percent sugar). Not only are these cereals bad for children's teeth, but the high level of sugar can cause blood sugar levels to rise quickly and then fall, leaving your child feeling tired and listless.

In an ideal world, our children would eat whole-grain cereals like muesli and oatmeal, and whole-grain bread, but even if your child is hooked on sugary cereals, she's still getting calcium from the milk she adds to the cereal (sugary cereals contain lots of carbohydrates). You might find that mixing sugary cereals with whole-grain cereals makes a good compromise. You can also boost the nutrition in a bowl of cereal by adding fresh or dried fruit, or try sprinkling cereals with wheat germ.

Healthy eating: *Chubby babies at the age of one soon slim down once they start walking.*

Fruit

Breakfast provides a good opportunity to eat some fresh fruit toward the recommended five portions of fruit and vegetables each day. Different fruits contain different vitamins, so try to include plenty of variety. Think of different ways of presenting fruit, like a two-color fruit salad, or cut a kiwi in half, serve it in an egg cup, and let your child scoop out the flesh with a teaspoon. Fruity milkshakes are another way to encourage your child to consume more fruit, or make fruit smoothies—mango, strawberry, banana, and fresh orange juice is a delicious combination.

Helping fussy children

Babies grow more rapidly in their first year than at any other time in their lives, but after twelve months, a child's growth and weight-gain generally slow down. It is not so surprising, therefore, that many children who were good eaters in their first year become more fussy, and the second year is often a time when food is used to assert independence.

Once your child starts to walk and to get around by himself, his life becomes much more interesting. Many toddlers lose interest in food around this stage and would much rather play with their toys and run around. However unreasonable your child's eating habits, try to respond calmly. Food shouldn't be used as a means to teach a child to do as he is told. If your child refuses his meal, don't make a fuss, but leave the meal in front of him and carry on eating your own meal. He will soon realize that refusing food isn't much fun when you don't react and he doesn't get the attention he is looking for. You need to be firm and consistent and try to make mealtimes enjoyable. Introduce your baby to a wide variety of foods; it's surprising how sophisticated their tastes can be at a very early age. Allow your child to taste food from your plate—someone else's food is often more tempting. Give your child lots of praise when he tries a new food.

Your baby's milk

At one year, children can switch from formula or breast milk to whole cow's milk. The iron in breast milk is easily absorbed and infant formulas also contain good quantities of iron. Cow's milk, however, is a poor source of iron and can also block iron absorption if given as part of a meal, so make sure that your child gets plenty of iron in her daily diet in other ways (see page 17).

From one year your child needs about 14 ounces of milk a day, but give full-fat cow's milk and not skimmed milk before the age of two, as the latter is low in the energy that your child needs to grow. For very picky eaters there may be advantages in continuing with a baby formula (which is fortified with vitamins and iron) until two years of age. Yogurts or pasteurized cheese can be used as equivalents to milk, and you can smuggle milk into recipes like cauliflower with cheese sauce or rice pudding.

Family cuisine

Life is too short to cook a different meal for every member of the family. At this age, toddlers can eat almost everything that adult members of the family eat, with the exception of whole nuts, unpasteurized soft cheeses, and lightly cooked eggs. This is a good time to review your family's eating habits, as it is important to set up a healthy eating pattern for your child very early on, rather than wait until they are three or four when they already have strong likes and dislikes. It is great if young children can eat regularly with the rest of the family where they can see a selection of foods being enjoyed.

Attractive presentation will help to make a meal appealing to a toddler. Without going to extremes, bright colors and interesting shapes can go a long way to stimulating a reluctant appetite. If you are making a recipe for the whole family, such as a shepherd's pie, it is much more attractive to prepare a mini portion in a small dish like a ramekin rather than dollop a spoonful onto your child's plate. It can save time to plan ahead and when cooking a recipe, make several small portions that can be frozen for future use. Most of the recipes in this book are suitable for freezing, and this is always indicated by the F symbol next to relevant recipes.

Meal planner

	BREAKFAST	LUNCH	SUPPER
DAY 1	Cereal Peach Melba Smoothie (page 111)	Rice 'n' Easy (page 106) Peach, Strawberry, and Raspberry Ice Pops (page 108)	Homemade Cream of Tomato Soup (page 94) Baked potato Fruit
DAY 2	French Toast (page 86) Fruit	Scarlett's Spaghetti Bolognese (page 104) Fruit	Rabbit Muffins (page 94) Yogurt and honey
DAY 3	Oatmeal Yogurt	Orzo Risotto (page 96) Fruit and ice cream	Gratin of Haddock with Tomato Sauce and Spinach (page 105) Fruit
DAY 4	Scrambled egg and toast Fruit	Meatballs with Sweet-and-sour Sauce (page 102) and Chinese Fried Rice (page 123) Lara's Luscious Lychee Ice Pops (page 108)	Brown Rice with Diced Vegetables (page 97) Fun Ways with Fruit (page 108)
DAY 5	Cereal Peach Melba Smoothie (page 111)	Annabel's Tasty Chicken Skewers (page 101) Rice and vegetables Summer Fruit Brûlée (page 111)	Tomato Sauce with Hidden Vegetables (page 99) Pasta Fruit
DAY 6	Cheese on toast Fruit	Fillet of Fish with Herb Butter (page 105) with vegetables and french fries Fruit	Carrot Soup with Yellow Split Peas (page 96) Baked potato Fresh Peach Melba (page 85)
DAY 7	Scrambled egg and toast Fruit	Cheese and Zucchini Sausages (page 100) Fruit	Chicken with Matchsticks (page 100) Peach, Strawberry, and Raspberry Ice Pops (page 108)

Three servings of dairy products should be included daily, such as cheese, yogurt, and a milk-based drink.

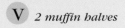

  5 portions

Tomatoes *are an excellent source of lycopene, an antioxidant pigment that helps to prevent cancer and heart disease. However, research shows that lycopene in tomatoes can be absorbed more efficiently by the body if the tomatoes have been cooked with a little oil.*

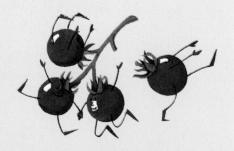

Rabbit muffins

1 pat unsalted butter
1 scallion, finely chopped
½ cup grated Cheddar cheese
1 whole-wheat English muffin,
   split in half
1 tablespoon good-quality tomato sauce

DECORATION
1 carrot
1 black olive
Frozen peas
Corn kernels
Sprouts

Melt the butter and sauté the scallion until softened. Stir in the grated cheese until melted. Toast the muffin halves and divide the tomato sauce between them, then cover with the cheese sauce. Cook under a preheated broiler until golden (about 2 minutes). If you like, decorate the muffin halves to look like rabbits.

Homemade cream of tomato soup

Some children don't like green bits floating around in their soup, so you can leave out the basil if your child prefers.

1½ tablespoons olive oil
1 medium onion, chopped
1 clove garlic, crushed
2 medium carrots, peeled and sliced
1 medium potato, peeled and diced
One 14.5-ounce can chopped tomatoes
1 pound plum tomatoes, peeled,
   seeded, and chopped

1 tablespoon tomato paste
¼ teaspoon superfine sugar
2 cups chicken or vegetable
   stock
Freshly ground black pepper
3 tablespoons heavy cream, light cream,
   or half-and-half (optional)
2 tablespoons torn fresh basil leaves
   (optional)

Warm the olive oil in a large pan over low heat, then add the onion and garlic and sauté for 2 to 3 minutes. Add the carrots and potato and sauté for about 8 minutes. Add the remaining ingredients, except for the cream and basil. Bring to a boil, then cover and simmer for about 30 minutes. Blend in a food processor until smooth and press through a sieve. Add the cream and basil (if using) and reheat, but do not bring to a boil.

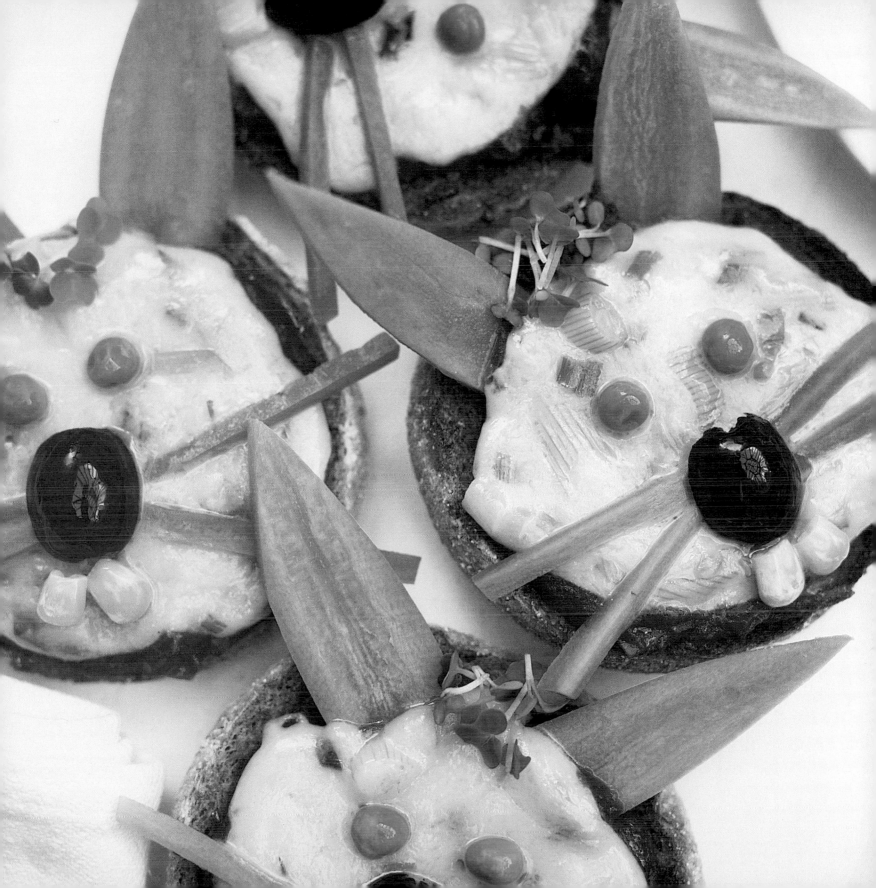

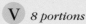
Carrots *do improve night vision. They are an excellent source of beta-carotene, which is converted in the body into vitamin A. One of the first symptoms of vitamin A deficiency is night blindness.*

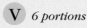 6 portions

Pasta *is a good source of complex carbohydrates, which provide us with sustained energy. This is why it is so popular with athletes. Try mixing some whole-grain pasta with regular pasta to increase the fiber content of the meal.*

Did you know?

Sixty percent of the energy in an adult's diet should come from carbohydrates.

Carrot soup with yellow split peas

This soup is packed full of nutrients and is a good source of protein for vegetarians.

1 cup yellow split peas

1 tablespoon unsalted butter

4 medium carrots, peeled and sliced

1 medium onion, chopped

1 bay leaf

1 clove garlic, crushed

$\frac{1}{2}$ cup washed and sliced white part of a leek

4 cups vegetable stock

2 tablespoons sour cream

1 tablespoon chopped fresh parsley

Salt and freshly ground black pepper

Soak the split peas in cold water overnight. Melt the butter in a large saucepan and sauté the carrots, onion, bay leaf, and garlic for 3 to 4 minutes. Stir in the leek and drained split peas. Pour in the vegetable stock, cover, bring to a boil, and simmer for 40 minutes. Remove the bay leaf and blend the soup in a food processor. Stir in the sour cream and parsley and season to taste.

Orzo risotto

1 tablespoon olive oil

2 tablespoons unsalted butter

1 medium onion, finely chopped

1 clove garlic, crushed

1 cup diced zucchini

$\frac{1}{2}$ red or yellow bell pepper, seeded and diced

$1\frac{1}{2}$ cups diced button mushrooms

$1\frac{1}{2}$ cups orzo or other small pasta shapes

1 teaspoon finely chopped fresh thyme

1 bay leaf

4 cups chicken or vegetable stock

$\frac{1}{4}$ cup freshly grated Parmesan cheese

Salt and freshly ground black pepper

Heat the oil and half the butter. Sauté the onion, garlic, and zucchini for 5 minutes. Stir in the bell pepper and mushrooms and sauté for 2 minutes. Stir in the orzo, thyme, bay leaf, and about a quarter of the stock and cook over low heat until the stock is almost absorbed, stirring frequently. Gradually add the rest of the stock, stirring each time, until almost all the liquid has been absorbed. This will take a total of about 20 minutes. Remove the bay leaf and stir in the remaining butter and the cheese. Season to taste.

Brown rice with diced vegetables

 6 portions

Personally, I have always liked the nutty taste of brown rice, and it is good to introduce it to your child so that he doesn't eat only ordinary white rice. You can substitute sliced mushrooms for the eggplant if you prefer, as some children aren't too keen on eggplant.

3 cups vegetable stock
1 cup brown rice
2 tablespoons olive oil
1 medium red onion, chopped
1 clove garlic, crushed
1 small red bell pepper, seeded and diced
1 zucchini, diced
½ small eggplant, diced
1 tablespoon tomato puree
¼ cup grated Parmesan cheese
Salt and freshly ground black pepper

Place the stock in a saucepan and bring to a boil. Add the rice, cover, and boil for 30 to 45 minutes or until tender and most of the stock has been absorbed. Remove the lid for the last 10 minutes. The mixture should resemble rice pudding in consistency.

In a separate pan, heat the olive oil. Sauté the onion and bell pepper for 7 minutes. Add the garlic and sauté for 1 minute more. Add the zucchini and eggplant and cook for an additional 8 minutes. Stir in the tomato puree and cook for 2 minutes. Stir in the cooked rice and cheese and season to taste.

BROWN RICE *provides a good source of energy, some protein, B vitamins, and minerals. It is much more nutritious to eat brown rice, as white rice has lost most of its important minerals and vitamins during processing. The starch in rice, particularly brown rice, is absorbed slowly, thereby providing a steady release of glucose for sustained energy. Brown rice is also a good source of fiber and potassium.*

Healthy eating: *There is always some nutrient loss when vegetables are cooked, particularly the water-soluble vitamins B and C. However, when vegetables are cooked in stock to make soup, the liquid absorbs the water-soluble vitamins and since we end up consuming both the liquid and the vegetables, more of the original nutrient content is retained.*

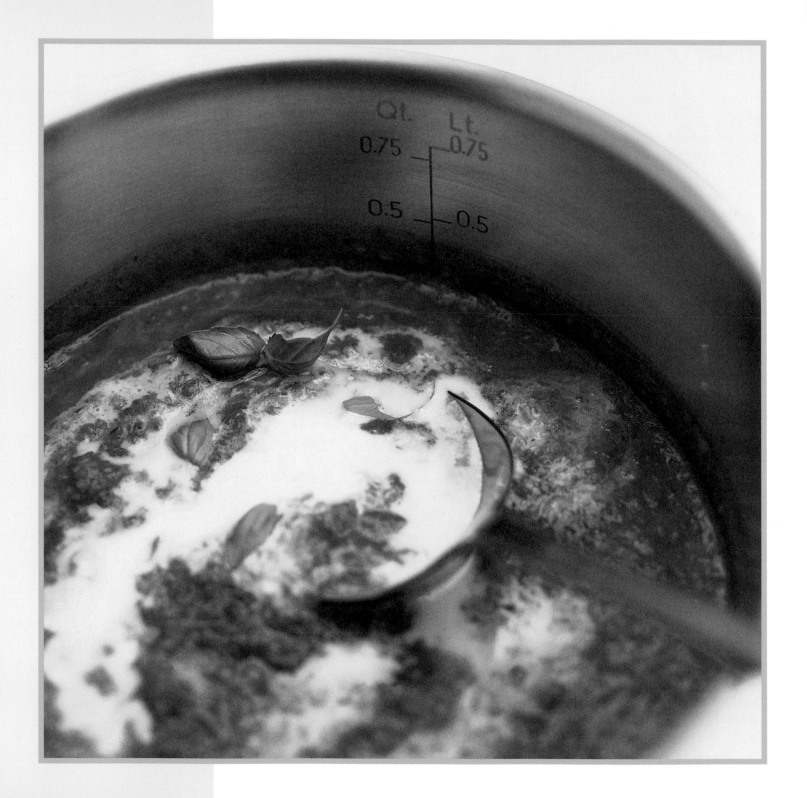

Tomato sauce with hidden vegetables

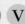

This is a delicious tomato sauce flavored, if you like, with a hint of creamy mascarpone cheese. This is a great way to get children to eat vegetables because the sauce makes the vegetables invisible—and what children can't see, they can't pick out. Serve with the pasta of your choice.

1 medium onion, chopped

1 clove garlic, crushed

1 tablespoon vegetable oil

1 large carrot, peeled and sliced

½ red bell pepper, seeded and diced

1 cup diced zucchini

2 tablespoons unsalted butter

½ white part of a leek, washed and sliced

1 cup chopped button mushrooms

3 plum tomatoes, peeled, seeded, and chopped

One 14 ounce can tomato puree

1 tablespoon torn fresh basil leaves

1 tablespoon chopped fresh parsley

Pinch of sugar

Salt and freshly ground black pepper

¼ cup mascarpone cheese (optional)

1½ cups pasta shapes

Sauté the onion and garlic in the oil until beginning to soften (about 2 minutes). Add the carrot and sauté for 4 minutes. Add the red pepper and zucchini and sauté until beginning to soften (2 to 3 minutes). Add the butter, leek, and mushrooms and cook for 5 minutes. Add the tomatoes, tomato puree, basil, parsley, sugar, and salt and pepper and simmer, covered, for 15 minutes. Blend in a food processor. Press through a sieve and stir in the mascarpone cheese, if using.

Meanwhile, cook the pasta according to the package instructions. When it's cooked, drain in a colander and toss with the tomato sauce.

Brightly colored vegetables *contain a wide variety of phytochemicals (plant chemicals) that will give us a greater chance of preventing diseases such as coronary heart disease and cancer. Canned tomatoes retain most of their nutrients but do also contain salt.*

SUPERFOODS

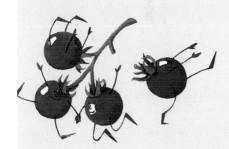

SUPERFOODS

Cheese *is particularly beneficial at the end of a meal, as it raises the calcium concentration in plaque. Protein from cheese is also absorbed onto the enamel surface of the teeth and physically slows down tooth decay.*

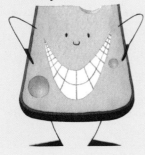

Cheese and zucchini sausages

Delicious vegetarian sausages are quick and easy to prepare. If you have time, you can form the mixture into sausage shapes and then set aside in the fridge to firm up before frying.

3 slices white bread
2 tablespoons unsalted butter
1 medium onion, finely chopped
1¼ cups grated zucchini

1 cup grated Cheddar cheese
1 egg, separated
A little salt and freshly ground black pepper
Vegetable oil for frying

Make bread crumbs by tearing the bread into pieces and blitzing it in a food processor.

Heat the butter in a frying pan and fry the onion until soft. Add the grated zucchini and cook for 3 minutes or until softened.

Mix with the grated cheese, half the bread crumbs, the egg yolk, and seasoning. Shape into 8 sausages about 4 inches long, using floured hands. Dip into the lightly beaten egg white and then roll in the remaining bread crumbs.

Heat some oil in a wok or frying pan and cook the sausages over medium heat, turning carefully as necessary, until lightly golden.

SUPERFOODS

Chicken *contains much less fat than other meats, as most of the fat lies in the skin, which can be removed. However, chicken with the skin on is higher in fat than beef and other red meats.*

Chicken with matchsticks

This is simple to make and everything is cut into little bite-size pieces perfect for a one-year-old. As a special treat you can buy child-friendly plastic chopsticks, which are joined at the top and can be used by children as young as two. Serve with rice.

SAUCE
2 teaspoons red wine vinegar
2 tablespoons soy sauce
2 tablespoons ketchup
2 tablespoons olive oil
¼ cup pineapple juice
2 teaspoons sugar

2 boneless, skinless chicken breasts,
    cut into strips
Salt and freshly ground black pepper
1½ tablespoons vegetable oil
¼ cup carrot matchsticks
¼ cup zucchini matchsticks (unpeeled)
2 pieces canned whole baby corn,
    sliced in half lengthwise

Mix together all the ingredients for the sauce and set aside. Season the chicken with a little salt and pepper and sauté in the oil until cooked through (4 to 5 minutes). Drain on paper towels. Steam the carrot, zucchini, and baby corn for about 4 minutes so that they are cooked but still crunchy. Bring the sauce to a boil, simmer for about a minute, and stir in the vegetable strips and chicken.

Annabel's tasty chicken skewers

Marinated chicken skewers make an easy-to-prepare and very tasty meal. They can also be cooked on the barbecue.

2 tablespoons soy sauce
¼ cup light brown sugar
1½ teaspoons lime or lemon juice
1½ teaspoons vegetable oil
½ small clove garlic, crushed
2 boneless, skinless chicken breasts, cut into chunks

Put the soy sauce and sugar into a small saucepan and gently heat until the sugar has dissolved. Remove from the heat; stir in the lime or lemon juice, vegetable oil, and garlic. Allow the marinade to cool for a few minutes and then marinate the chicken for at least 1 hour or overnight in the refrigerator. Soak four bamboo skewers in water to prevent them from getting scorched. Preheat the oven to 350°F. Thread the chunks of chicken onto the skewers, place on a baking sheet lined with foil, and bake for 6 to 7 minutes per side, basting occasionally with the marinade until cooked through.

4 portions

Chicken *is an excellent source of lean protein and is very versatile. It might be a good idea in this recipe to make skewers using chicken breast and chicken thigh together, as the dark meat of the chicken contains twice as much iron and zinc as the light meat.*

SUPERFOODS

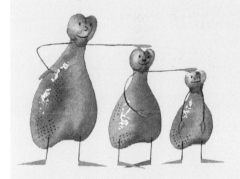

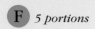
SUPERFOODS

Red meat *contains iron that is more easily absorbed than iron in fruit, vegetables, grains, and eggs. However, meat will help to boost the absorption of iron from vegetables and cereals when eaten at the same time.*

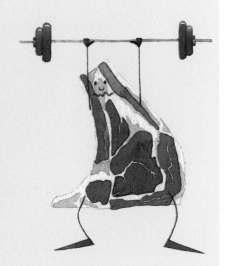

Meatballs with sweet-and-sour sauce

These miniature meatballs are made with lean beef in a very tasty tomato-flavored sweet-and-sour sauce and served with Chinese Fried Rice (see page 123). This is a great favorite with all my family.

MEATBALLS

1 pound lean ground beef

1 medium onion, finely chopped

1 apple, peeled and grated

$\frac{1}{2}$ cup fresh white bread crumbs

1 tablespoon chopped fresh parsley

1 chicken bouillon cube, finely crumbled

2 tablespoons cold water

Salt and freshly ground black pepper

2 tablespoons vegetable oil

SWEET-AND-SOUR SAUCE

1 tablespoon soy sauce

$1\frac{1}{2}$ teaspoons cornstarch

1 tablespoon vegetable oil

1 medium onion, finely chopped

$\frac{1}{4}$ cup diced red bell pepper

One 14.5-ounce can chopped tomatoes

1 tablespoon cider vinegar

1 teaspoon brown sugar

Freshly ground black pepper

Mix together all the ingredients for the meatballs and chop for a few seconds in a food processor. Using floured hands, form into about 20 meatballs. Heat the oil in a frying pan and sauté the meatballs, turning occasionally, until browned and sealed (10 to 12 minutes).

Meanwhile, to make the sauce, mix together the soy sauce and cornstarch in a small bowl. Heat the oil in a pan and sauté the onion for 3 minutes. Add the bell pepper and sauté, stirring occasionally, for 2 minutes. Add the tomatoes, vinegar, and sugar, season with pepper, and simmer for 10 minutes. Add the soy sauce mixture and cook for 2 minutes, stirring occasionally. Blend and strain, or puree the sauce through a food mill. Pour the sauce over the meatballs, cover, and simmer until heated through (about 5 minutes). Serve with fried rice.

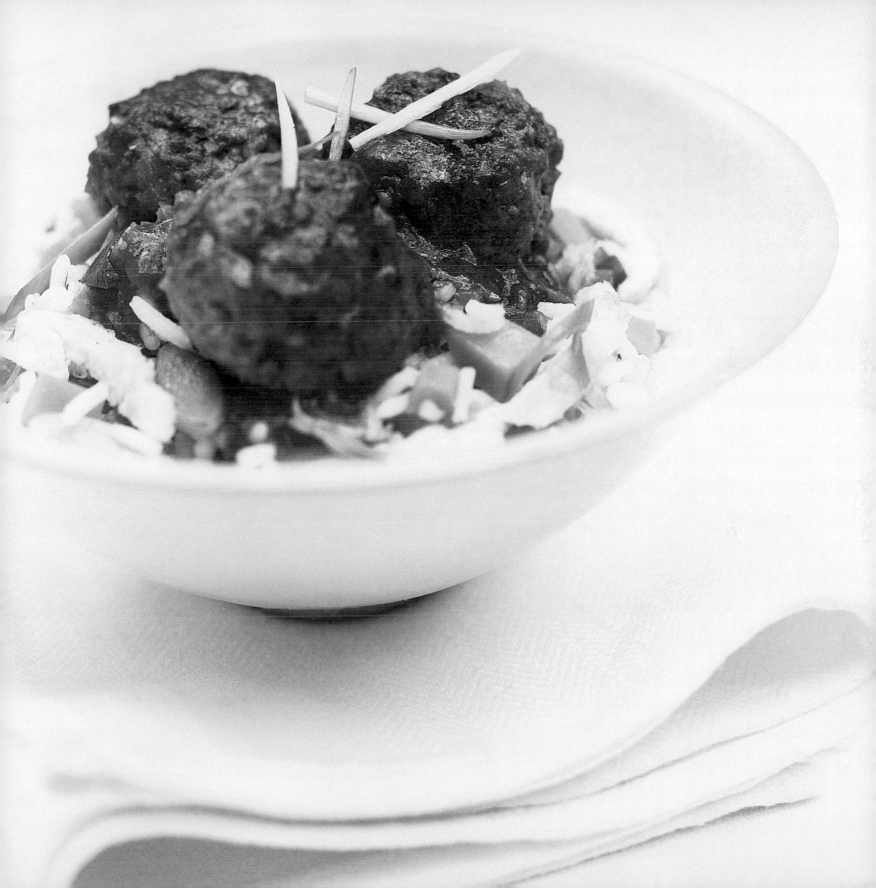

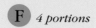

F *4 portions*

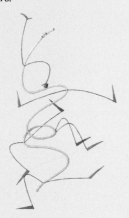

SUPERFOODS

Red meat *is best included in your child's diet two or three times a week, as it is the best source of readily absorbed iron. Iron requirements rise when the body is growing fast; so it is especially important to make sure your child gets enough iron between 6 months and 2 years.*

Scarlett's spaghetti Bolognese

This very tasty Bolognese sauce has hidden vegetables blended into it. My daughter Scarlett loves this recipe. Like so many children, she would be happy to eat pasta every day!

2 tablespoons vegetable oil

1 cup finely chopped onion

1 clove garlic, crushed

1 medium carrot, peeled and grated

1 cup sliced button mushrooms

1 beef bouillon cube dissolved in
   1 cup boiling water

8 ounces ground lean beef

6 tablespoons tomato puree

1 tablespoon ketchup

1½ teaspoons Worcestershire sauce

1 teaspoon brown sugar

1 bay leaf

1½ teaspoons cornstarch dissolved in
   2 tablespoons cold water

Salt and freshly ground black pepper

8 ounces spaghetti

Heat the oil in a saucepan, add the onion, and sauté for 6 to 7 minutes over low heat until softened, stirring occasionally. Add the crushed garlic and sauté for a few seconds.

Transfer half the onion to another saucepan. Add the carrot and mushrooms and cook for 3 minutes. Transfer to a blender, add half the beef stock, and blitz until smooth.

Add the ground beef to the remaining sautéed onion in the saucepan and cook, stirring occasionally, for 4 minutes or until browned. Add the remaining stock, the tomato puree, ketchup, Worcestershire sauce, brown sugar, and bay leaf. Stir in the carrot and mushroom puree and simmer, covered, for 9 minutes. Remove the bay leaf. Stir in the dissolved cornstarch, bring to a boil, and cook, stirring, for 1 minute. Add salt and pepper to taste. Cook the spaghetti according to the package instructions. Drain in a colander and toss with the Bolognese sauce.

Fillet of fish with herb butter

2 tablespoons softened unsalted butter

2 tablespoons chopped mixed fresh herbs,
   such as parsley, thyme, oregano, and basil

1 tablespoon lemon juice

1 pound thick cod fillets, skinned

Coarse sea salt and freshly ground
   black pepper

Preheat the oven to 350°F. Mix the butter with the herbs and lemon juice. Place the fish in a small ovenproof dish, season with salt and pepper, and spread the herb butter over the top. Bake until the fish is cooked through (8 to 10 minutes). Flake with a fork, checking to make sure there are no bones. Delicious with creamy mashed potatoes and peas.

Gratin of haddock with tomato sauce and spinach

Once cooked, the fish will just flake with a fork and be nice and soft for your baby to eat.

1 tablespoon olive oil

½ cup finely chopped onion

1 small clove garlic, crushed

1 cup canned chopped tomatoes

1½ teaspoons tomato puree

½ teaspoon sugar

8 ounces fresh spinach, washed and
   tough stems removed

10 ounces haddock or other
   white fish fillets, skinned

2 tablespoons all-purpose flour

2 tablespoons unsalted butter

½ cup grated Cheddar cheese

Preheat the oven to 350°F. Heat the oil in a saucepan and sauté the onion for 5 minutes. Add the garlic and sauté for 1 minute. Add the tomatoes, puree, and sugar, and simmer, covered, for 7 minutes. Cook the wet spinach leaves in a pan over medium heat for 3 minutes until just limp, then squeeze out the remaining moisture and chop coarsely. Coat the fish fillets in the flour, melt the butter in a small frying pan, and sauté the fish for about 1½ minutes on each side or until lightly golden and sealed. Spread the spinach over the base of a suitable ovenproof dish. Lay the fillets of fish on top, pour over the tomato sauce, and sprinkle with the grated cheese. Bake in the oven for 10 minutes or until the fish is cooked through. Flake the fish with a fork and mix together with the spinach and tomato and cheese sauce.

 2 to 3 portions

Herbs *have many medicinal properties. Parsley contains vitamin C and iron, and chewing on parsley is a good breath freshener, especially after eating garlic. Chewing thyme is thought to help soothe sore throats, and oregano as an infusion is thought to aid digestion and relieve cold symptoms.*

 4 servings

White fish *such as haddock and cod are an excellent source of low-fat protein and contain selenium, calcium, and magnesium. Eating fish helps fight free radicals and also boosts the immune system.*

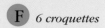 *6 croquettes*

Salmon *provides a good source of essential fats that support brain function and the immune system. Indeed, it is thought that the essential fatty acids in oily fish may help children who suffer from dyslexia or dyspraxia. An oily fish such as salmon should be included in all of our diets at least once a week.*

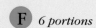 *6 portions*

Rice *contains starch that is digested and absorbed slowly, which provides a steady blood sugar level for long-lasting energy.*

Easy salmon croquettes

These salmon croquettes are really delicious and can be prepared in 10 minutes using pantry ingredients. They make good finger food and can also be eaten cold.

One 7.5-ounce can red salmon
1 heaping tablespoon grated or finely chopped onion
2 tablespoons ketchup
1 tablespoon fine matzo meal or fresh bread crumbs, plus extra for coating
2 tablespoons vegetable oil

Flake the salmon, checking carefully that there are no large bones and thoroughly mashing in the small, soft ones. In a mixing bowl, combine the salmon, onion, ketchup, and the 1 tablespoon of matzo meal or bread crumbs. Form into 6 small croquettes and coat in matzo meal or bread crumbs. Heat the oil in a frying pan and sauté the croquettes until golden (1 to 2 minutes per side).

Rice 'n' easy

A delicious, easy-to-prepare dish of cooked rice and tender pieces of chicken in a tasty tomato sauce. Rice tends to be very popular with young children and these are good textures to encourage your child to chew.

1 cup long-grain rice
1 tablespoon vegetable oil
1 large shallot or 1 small onion, chopped
½ small red bell pepper, seeded and chopped
1 tablespoon chopped fresh parsley
8 ounces boneless, skinless chicken breasts, chopped

2 cups tomato puree
1 chicken bouillon cube dissolved in ½ cup boiling water
1 clove garlic, finely chopped
1 teaspoon superfine sugar
Salt and freshly ground black pepper

Cook the rice according to the package instructions. While the rice is cooking, heat the oil in a large saucepan and sauté the shallot, red pepper, and parsley for about 5 minutes. Add the chopped chicken and sauté, stirring occasionally, until it turns opaque. Add the tomato puree, chicken stock, garlic, and sugar and season with salt and pepper. Cook, uncovered, for 15 minutes. Mix the cooked rice with the tomato sauce.

Oven-fried root vegetables

These make a great-tasting finger food. You can also use other root vegetables like carrots. They are very good served with a little bowl of sour cream and chive dip. For babies under a year, leave out the salt and seasoning.

1 medium potato, scrubbed
1 small sweet potato, scrubbed
1 small parsnip, scrubbed
1 tablespoon olive oil, plus extra for brushing the pan
All-purpose spicy seasoning such as Jane's Krazy Mixed-Up Salt or Old Bay Seasoning
Sea salt

DIP
4 ounces cream cheese
1½ teaspoons ketchup
1½ teaspoons whole milk
1 teaspoon snipped chives

Preheat the oven to 400°F. Cut the potato and sweet potato in half lengthwise and then into wedges about 1 inch thick. Cut the parsnip lengthwise into wedges. Put all the pieces into a bowl and toss with the olive oil, a sprinkling of seasoning, and a little salt (for babies over a year). Brush a roasting pan with a little olive oil and arrange the vegetable wedges in the pan. Bake until tender (about 30 minutes).

For the dip, mix together the cream cheese, ketchup, and milk and stir in the snipped chives. Serve with the vegetable wedges.

Sweet potatoes *are high in vitamins A and C and a particularly rich source of phytochemicals, which can help protect against disease.*

SUPERFOODS

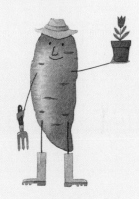

Citus and berry fruits *are a good source of vitamin C, which helps the absorption of iron from other foods, so try to give some vitamin C-rich fruits at every meal.*

 8 ice pops

Raspberries *contain ellagic acid, which can help protect us against cancer. Of all the fruits, raspberries pack the most fiber into the fewest calories.*

 6 ice pops

Lychees *are a good way to get some sweetness in the diet. They are also a good source of fiber and vitamins.*

Fun ways with fruit

It is fun to arrange fruit in novelty shapes and takes only a few minutes—and your child will probably want to give you a helping hand. Here, the fish is made from kiwifruit, orange, mango, nectarine, and grapes. Let your imagination run free and set about creating your dream house, a car, a boat—whatever you or your child comes up with. Different fruits contain different vitamins and minerals, so the more variety the better.

Peach, strawberry, and raspberry ice pops

If there is one food that almost no child can resist, it has to be an ice pop. Most of the pops you buy are full of sugar and artificial colors and flavor, but it takes very little time to make your own using good natural ingredients like pureed fresh fruit and fresh fruit juices. Small plastic or paper cups work wonderfully for making ice pops. You can also use empty yogurt containers.

6 strawberries, hulled
1 cup raspberries
1/3 cup confectioners' sugar, or to taste
2 cups peach juice

Puree the strawberries and raspberries and push through a sieve. Stir in the sugar until dissolved. Mix the fruit puree with the peach juice and pour into ice pop molds.

Lara's luscious lychee ice pops

One 20-ounce can lychees, or 2 cups lychee juice
1 tablespoon lemon juice

Blend the lychees together with the juice from the can and strain. Stir in the lemon juice and pour into ice pop molds.

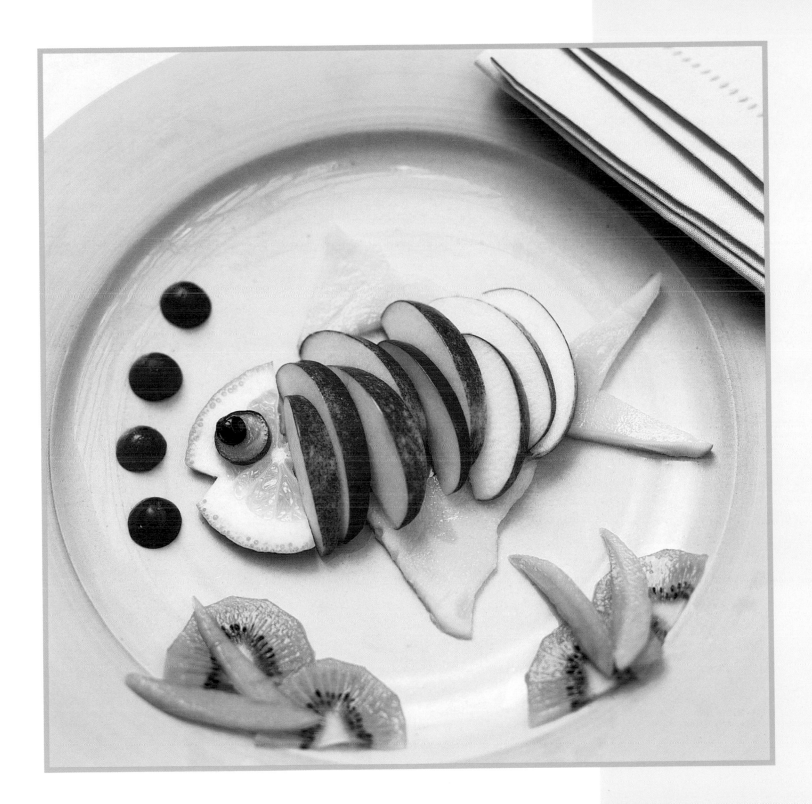

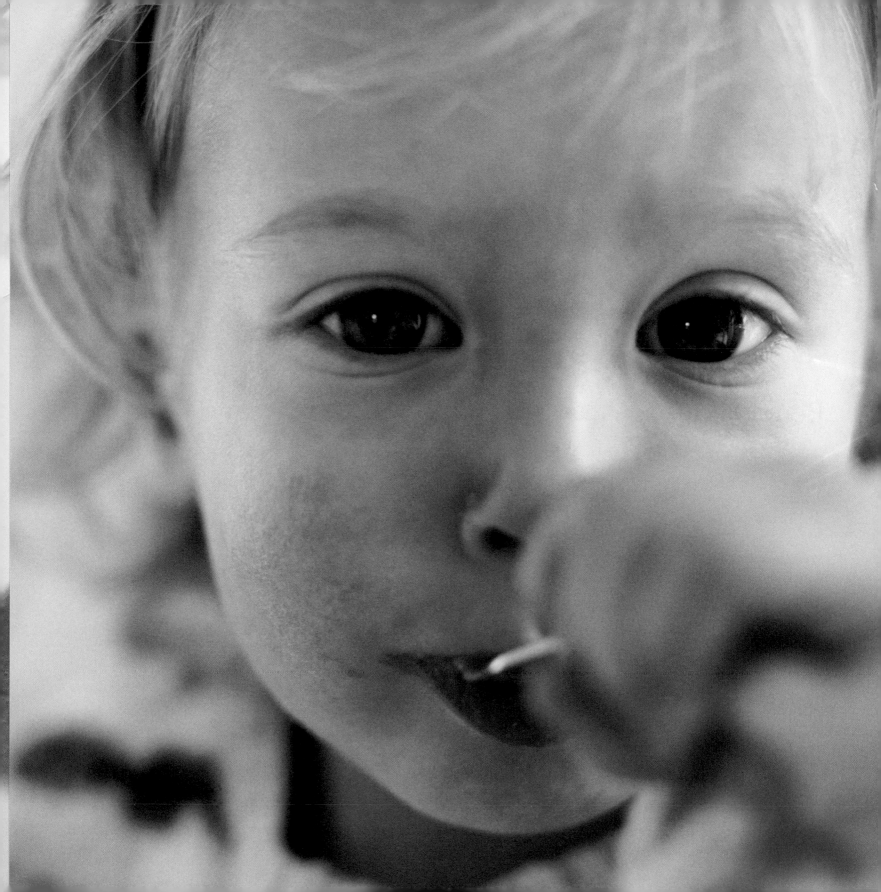

2 to 3 years:
SuperFoods for the growing years

Your child should now be enjoying a full and varied diet, and you should be able to cook meals for the whole family to enjoy. Make sure you offer plenty of healthy snacks, as many toddlers prefer lots of small meals to three big ones.

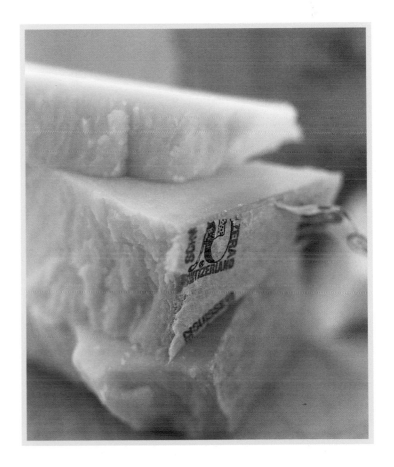

Healthy snacks

Young children require a large amount of energy in comparison to their body size, but they cannot cope with large quantities of food at any one time. Some toddlers may survive quite happily on three meals a day, but you will probably find that your child will also need snacks between meals to keep up her energy level. As babies become increasingly mobile and expend a lot of energy, it is important that you have plenty of healthy snacks on hand rather than let her fill herself up on empty calories like cookies and potato chips. Offer healthy snacks like cheese and dried or fresh fruit, or sandwiches with nutritious fillings like peanut butter or protein-based salads.

Young children have to eat concentrated sources of energy and nutrients frequently. It's a good idea to keep a stock of foods that lend themselves to snacks but that are wholesome and will give a child a slow release of energy. This is preferable to a faster boost of energy followed by a more rapid drop in blood sugars, as happens when sugary snacks are eaten.

Offer your child nutritious snacks like fruit or raw vegetables with a dip. It is regular snacking on sugary foods and drinks that does the most damage to children's teeth, so it is important to train young children to enjoy eating healthy snacks like the ones listed to the right.

You can aim toward a pattern of three meals a day, but it will probably take a few years for toddlers to get there. Toddlers have

Healthy eating: *Allow snacks only if there is more than an hour before the next meal so that children will still be hungry at mealtimes. Also try to restrict snacks to at least an hour after the last meal so that children don't get the idea that they can refuse a meal and then get something else to eat shortly afterward.*

Healthy eating: *Potato chips and tortilla chips are all right as part of a balanced diet, but choose a variety made with natural ingredients (vegetable chips are good) and preferably low salt. Limit your child to three small bags a week. Homemade popcorn is lower in fat and higher in fiber than potato chips and similar snacks.*

small tummies and often can't eat enough at one meal to be sustained through to the next. Be prepared to offer your toddler healthy between-meal snacks during the day. So many of us will die from diet-related diseases that setting up a good diet in the vital first few years may well determine your child's health later in life.

Some ideas for healthy snacks

- Fresh or dried fruit.
- Mini sandwiches.
- Yogurt.
- Whole-grain breakfast cereals.
- Steamed or raw vegetable sticks.
- Fingers of toast with honey or whole fruit spreads.
- Pita bread fingers and hummus.
- Rice cakes or sesame seed crackers.
- English muffins.
- Grilled cheese.
- Cheese.
- Cream cheese with mini bread sticks.
- A bowl of homemade soup or fresh soup from a carton.

Energy-rich snacks

Toddlers are usually very active and except at mealtimes will need good healthy snacks to keep up their energy. Toddlers tend to need frequent small meals. Unrefined carbohydrate foods like whole-wheat bread, whole-grain cereal, and potatoes take longer to break down into glucose and will provide a more nutritious and sustained energy supply than sugar and carbohydrates from refined sources like white bread and chocolate chip cookies. Fresh fruit also provides a good fast-working supply of energy.

Healthy junk food

There is no such thing as junk food, only a junk diet! Hamburgers, fries, potato chips, and chocolate eaten in moderation provide energy, protein, and even minerals like calcium. But it is now clear that a junk diet that is high in fat, sugar, and salt leads to health problems like obesity, heart disease, and cancer later on in life. Bad habits start very early on in life, so setting a good example by eating healthy foods will help protect your child's future.

Of course, fried foods are not bad for children, as the fat they use as energy to grow isn't related to any increased heart problems, and vegetable oils are better than animal fats. But fried foods must be only part of a healthy diet because, like anything else, too great an amount of fried food can be bad for children.

Good foods for a quick spurt of energy
- Bowl of cornflakes.
- Banana.
- Raisins.
- Yogurt and fruit with honey.

Good food for sustained energy
- Peanut butter on whole-wheat bread.
- Granola bar.
- Potato skins with cheese.
- Bread with ham, tuna, or cheese.
- Fresh fruit milkshake.

Foods like burgers and pizza tend to be very appealing, and children may well resent not being allowed to eat them, particularly if their friends get to eat them. However, a good solution is to prepare foods that look like the foods they want but are actually made from good healthy ingredients. Try Rabbit Muffins (page 94), Oven-Fried Root Vegetables (page 107), and Delicious Chicken Burgers with four different vegetables (page 128).

Obesity in children

The percentage of overweight children in the United States is growing at an alarming rate. Thirteen percent of children six to eleven years old are obese, as are 15 percent of children twelve to nineteen. If a child is obese at six, there is a 50 percent chance of lifelong obesity; if obese at thirteen, there is a 75 percent chance. Overweight children are more at risk for heart disease and stroke, and obesity doubles a child's risk of type 2 diabetes. Apart from ill health, overweight children are more likely to have poor self-esteem and to feel lonely.

Any parent who has tried to pry a child off the couch or away from the computer to go outside and play will know that children are becoming increasingly sedentary, more often than not moving nothing but a few fingers on a remote control. In fact, the problem has increased with the rise of technology and the proliferation of unhealthy convenience foods for children. Today our children tend to rely on cars rather than walking, video games and TV rather than outdoor play and exercise, and unhealthy and processed food rather than healthy, fresh choices.

The key to keeping children of all ages at a healthy weight is taking a family approach. Make healthy eating and exercise a family affair. Cut down on TV and computer games, and discourage eating while watching TV. Serve healthy meals and, whenever possible, eat meals together. Try to include five servings of fruit and vegetables a day. Plan healthy snacks and encourage children to eat a healthy breakfast.

Encourage children to be active, whether it is an organized soccer game, in-line skating, or going for a bike ride. Physical activity builds up muscle strength and overall fitness and develops important physical skills like balance and coordination. Children who develop an active lifestyle and are introduced to a variety of physical activities are much more likely to continue that healthy lifestyle in adulthood.

Helping to overcome obesity

The fatty deposits that lead to heart disease can already be found in the arteries of preschool children, and adult-onset diabetes—the type that normally affects middle-aged people—is already becoming a growing problem for kids in America. The number of

Other ways to help children who are overweight

• Set a good example by eating healthily yourself—don't expect your child to learn smart habits if you don't practice them yourself.

• Serve water or sugar-free soft drinks instead of fruit juice or sugary drinks.

• Cut out high-calorie between-meal snacks like potato chips or chocolate cookies and instead offer foods such as fruit, yogurts, or even a low-fat sandwich.

• It helps to serve meals on smaller plates to give the impression that portions are larger, and don't let children watch television or have other distractions while eating. Do not encourage more than one serving.

• Focus on more activity rather than less food.

• Make fitness fun.

• Charbroiling food on a ridged pan is a tasty, low-fat way to prepare chicken, fish, and meat.

What your toddler should be eating daily

Serving sizes will vary according to age and the individual child. However, this can be used as a rough guide for a two-year-old.

• 3 to 4 servings carbohydrates, such as a slice of bread, a small bowl of cereal, and a small baked potato.

• 3 to 4 servings fruit and vegetables, such as an apple, a banana, a clementine, a carrot, and broccoli florets.

• 3 servings milk and dairy products, such as a glass of milk, a serving of yogurt, and a small portion of macaroni and cheese or cauliflower with cheese.

• 1 serving animal protein, such as 2 ounces lean meat, poultry, or fish or 1 egg, or 2 servings vegetable protein, such as tofu, legumes, or nuts, 2 ounces baked beans, or a peanut butter sandwich.

obese six- to seven-year-olds has doubled in the last ten years. If you are concerned about your child's weight, you should consult your pediatrician.

Unlike adults, overweight children should not be put on a restricted diet. Children are still growing and it is important that they eat a balanced, varied diet that provides adequate energy and protein as well as essential nutrients such as calcium and iron.

Instead, by adopting a long-term approach to healthy eating, it should be possible to ensure that a child's weight keeps pace with his increasing height. It is better by far to adopt a healthier eating plan rather than cutting down on the amount of food offered. No child should ever go hungry. Base a child's diet on the guidelines given on pages 13 to 18.

A child should feel loved and not judged—focus on health rather than appearance. Overweight children know they are fat. Attacking the weight itself could push a child to turn even more to food as emotional sustenance.

Meal planner

	BREAKFAST	LUNCH	SUPPER
DAY 1	Cereal Thinly sliced cheese Fruit	Delicious Chicken Burgers (page 128) with vegetables and fries Fruit	Cheat's Cheese Soufflé (page 133) Fruity Gelatin (page 140)
DAY 2	Scrambled egg with toast Fruit	Vegetable Croquettes (page 134) Traffic Light Ice Pops (page 146)	Singapore Stir-fried Noodles (page 130) Summer Fruit Brûlée (page 111)
DAY 3	Oatmeal Yogurt and honey	Special Tomato Pasta Sauce (page 118) Pasta Fruit	Chicken and Broccoli Salad (page 124) Strawberry and Rhubarb Crumble (page 140) with custard sauce
DAY 4	Cereal with chopped dried fruit Unsweetened applesauce Yogurt	Bow-tie Pasta with Salmon and Tomatoes (page 139) Fruit	Beef in Hoisin Sauce with Broccoli and Water Chestnuts (page 129)
DAY 5	Boiled egg with fingers of toast Fruit Smoothies (page 143)	Marinated Chicken and Vegetables on a Griddle (page 120) Fruit	Spinach and Ricotta Cannelloni (page 127) Fruity Gelatin (page 140)
DAY 6	Cheese and tomato on toast Fruit	Fish and Chips in a Comic (page 137) Traffic Light Ice Pops (page 146)	Chicken Salad with Corn, Pasta, and Cherry Tomatoes (page 118) Strawberry and Rhubarb Crumble (page 140)
DAY 7	Pancake/waffle and maple syrup Yogurt and fruit	Cheesy Baked Potato with Butternut Squash (page 132) Fruit and ice cream	Sweet-and-sour Turkey Balls (page 125) with rice Peach Melba Frozen Yogurt with Crushed Meringues (page 145)

Include three servings of dairy products daily, such as cheese, yogurt, and a milk-based drink.

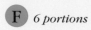
Chicken salad with corn, pasta, and cherry tomatoes

2 boneless, skinless chicken breasts
2½ cups chicken stock
½ cup pasta shapes, cooked and cooled
1 cup canned or cooked frozen corn
18 cherry tomatoes, cut in half
2 scallions, finely sliced
½ head Boston, Bibb, or romaine lettuce, shredded

DRESSING
3 tablespoons olive oil
1 tablespoon white wine vinegar
½ teaspoon Dijon mustard
½ teaspoon sugar
Salt and freshly ground black pepper
1 tablespoon of the stock used to poach the chicken

Put the chicken into a saucepan and cover with the stock. Bring to a boil, then cook over low heat (barely simmering) for about 20 minutes or until the chicken is cooked through. Let cool completely, remove with a slotted spoon, and cut into bite-size pieces. This can be done the night before. To make the dressing, whisk together all of the ingredients (or use a handheld blender). Mix together all the salad ingredients and toss in the dressing.

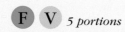
Special tomato pasta sauce

2 red bell peppers, seeded and cut into wide strips
1 shallot, finely chopped
1 small clove garlic, crushed
1 tablespoon olive oil

4 medium tomatoes, peeled, seeded, and roughly chopped
1 cup vegetable stock
1 tablespoon butter
Salt and freshly ground black pepper

Roast the red peppers under a preheated broiler until the skin is charred. Place the peppers in a plastic bag and seal. Set aside to cool down a little. Meanwhile, sauté the shallot and garlic in the olive oil until softened but not colored. Add the tomatoes and cook for 5 minutes. Remove the skin from the roasted peppers (it should come away easily) and add the peppers to the sauce together with the vegetable stock. Cook over low heat for about 10 minutes. Stir in the butter, puree in a food processor, and season to taste. Serve as a sauce for cooked pasta. The sauce is also very good served with chicken.

Crispy cheese, cabbage, and potato bake

 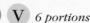

This tasty, thinly sliced potato gratin makes a delicious meal on a cold day together with something like a bowl of soup. It would also make a delicious accompaniment to a family meal. This dish was inspired by the Irish dish Colcannon, a hearty one-pot dinner of potatoes and cabbage.

1 tablespoon butter

1 large or 2 medium onions, very thinly sliced

½ cup light cream

1½ pounds potatoes, peeled and thinly sliced

1 cup shredded green cabbage

Salt and freshly ground black pepper

¾ cup grated Cheddar cheese

¾ cup grated Swiss cheese

1¼ cups whole milk

Preheat the oven to 350°F. Melt the butter in a saucepan over low heat and cook the onion until softened. Cover the bottom of an 8-inch square baking pan with a thin layer of cream, then with a layer of one-third of the potatoes and cabbage sprinkled with salt and pepper. Spoon one-third of the onion on top. Mix together the cheeses and sprinkle one-third of the mixture over the onion.

Continue with two more layers of potato, cabbage, onion, and cheese. Mix the milk together with the remaining cream and pour over the potato mixture. Cover with foil and bake for 30 minutes, then bake, uncovered, for about 30 minutes more or until golden and crispy on top. Test with a knife to make sure the potatoes are soft.

Green cabbage *is rich in beta-carotene and vitamin C. Cabbage belongs to the crucifer family, whose protective powers against cancer have been demonstrated in many studies. The phytochemicals in cabbage were once thought to be poisonous to humans. It also contains antioxidants that fight coronary heart disease by mopping up free radicals.*

SUPERFOODS

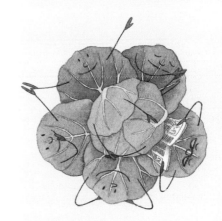

Monounsaturated
oils *such as olive oil can help to lower blood cholesterol levels. Interestingly, there is a lower incidence of cancer in Mediterranean countries where they use lots of olive oil. Olive oil is also a good source of vitamin E. Extra-virgin olive oil contains the highest quantity of protective antioxidants and has the best flavor.*

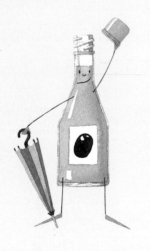

Marinated chicken and vegetables on a griddle

Cooking food on a griddle is a very healthy way of cooking, as it uses very little fat. Marinating the chicken before cooking it gives it a wonderful flavor and makes it nice and tender. Make sure the griddle is very hot before you lay the food on it.

1 large new potato, scrubbed and cut in half

3 broccoli florets

½ red bell pepper, seeded and cut into strips

2 boneless, skinless chicken breasts

1 zucchini

1 medium red onion

MARINADE

1 clove garlic, crushed

2 to 3 tablespoons lemon juice

¼ teaspoon grated lemon zest

1 teaspoon superfine sugar

1 teaspoon chopped fresh oregano or thyme

Salt and freshly ground black pepper

3 tablespoons olive oil

Parboil the potato for about 10 minutes. Blanch the broccoli and red pepper for 1 minute. Thinly slice the chicken breasts into about four pieces each. Cover the slices with plastic wrap and flatten with a mallet or rolling pin until about ¼ inch thick. Wash and cut the zucchini into ½-inch slices and cut the onion into six to eight wedges.

For the marinade, mix together the garlic, lemon juice and zest, sugar, and oregano or thyme, and add salt and pepper to taste. Stir the chicken into the marinade together with the vegetables and leave to marinate for about 30 minutes.

Heat a griddle (or you can use a frying pan), brush with a little of the olive oil, and remove the chicken from the marinade and cook for about 3 minutes on each side or until cooked through. Remove and keep warm. Repeat the same process with the vegetables, adding more olive oil if necessary, and cooking in batches if necessary. Mix the chicken and vegetables together and serve.

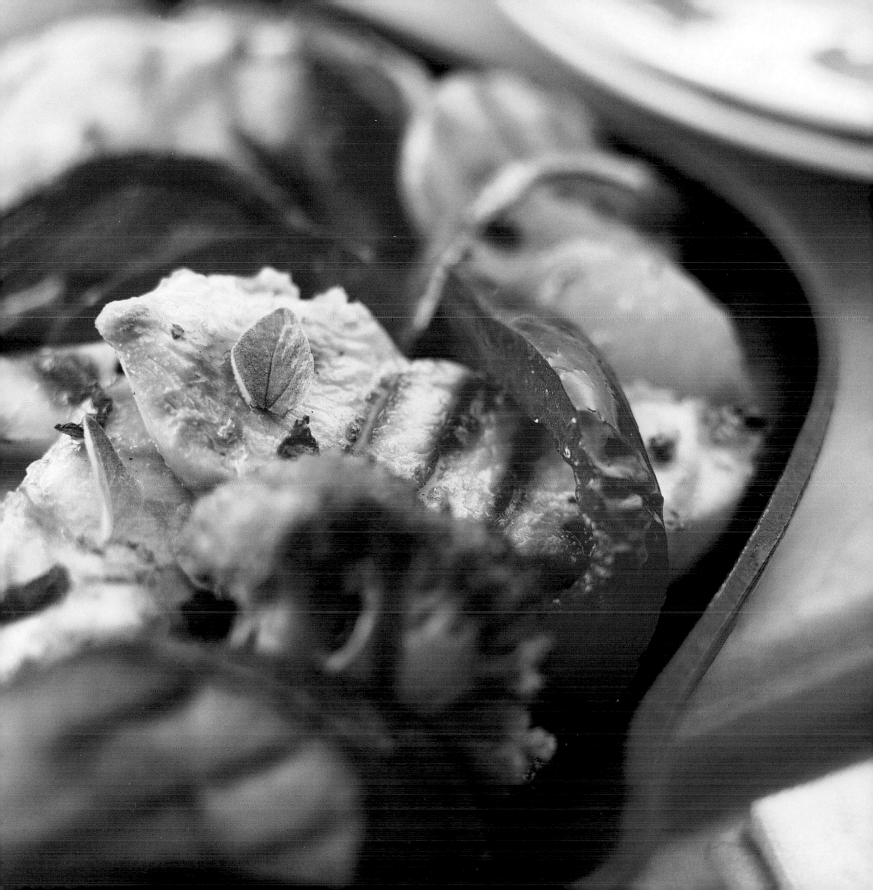

SUPERFOODS

Cheese *is a good source of protein and also provides calcium for the growth of healthy bones and teeth. Calcium in dairy products is more easily absorbed by the body than from other foods. Cheese is also a source of tryptophan, an amino acid that the body converts into serotonin, which makes us feel happy and in a good mood.*

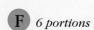

SUPERFOODS

Garlic *has the reputation of a cure-all in folk medicine and has been proven to help develop resistance to infection. Garlic contains allicin, which acts as a natural antibiotic and antifungal, and it is also high in antioxidants. Worshiped by the ancient Egyptians, chewed by Greek athletes, and essential for keeping vampires at bay, garlic is also good for zapping bacteria, maintaining a healthy heart, and warding off colds.*

Annabel's chicken dippers

Very yummy and a great favorite with my children. These are good served with ketchup.

2 boneless, skinless chicken breasts
¼ cup grated Parmesan cheese
¼ cup grated Cheddar cheese
¼ cup bread crumbs
½ teaspoon paprika
¼ to ½ teaspoon cayenne pepper

Salt and freshly ground black pepper
1 egg, lightly beaten
2 tablespoons all-purpose flour

6 tablespoons vegetable oil

Cut each chicken breast into ½-inch-wide strips. Mix together the Parmesan, Cheddar, bread crumbs, paprika, and cayenne, and add salt and pepper to taste. Place the beaten egg in a shallow dish, the flour in another, and the bread crumb mixture in a third. Dip each chicken strip first into the flour, then into the egg, and finally coat with the crumb mixture.

Heat the oil in a frying pan and fry the breaded chicken strips in batches over medium heat, taking care not to crowd the pan. Sauté until golden, about 2 minutes per side, then drain on paper towels.

Drumsticks with barbecue sauce

A very tasty way to prepare drumsticks.

6 chicken drumsticks

MARINADE
3 tablespoons ketchup
1 tablespoon vegetable oil
1 tablespoon rice wine vinegar

1 tablespoon soy sauce
2 tablespoons honey
1 teaspon paprika
1 clove garlic, crushed

Wash the drumsticks, pat dry with paper towels, and score each drumstick three times using a sharp knife. Thoroughly combine all the ingredients for the marinade. Coat the drumsticks in the marinade and refrigerate for 30 minutes or overnight.

Preheat the oven to 400°F. Line a baking tray or roasting pan with foil. Place the drumsticks in the pan together with the marinade. Roast for 35 to 40 minutes or until the chicken is thoroughly cooked.

Chinese fried rice

This is very popular with children and makes a good accompaniment to the Sweet-and-sour Turkey Balls on page 125 or Meatballs with Sweet-and-sour Sauce (page 102).

1 cup basmati rice
1 medium carrot, peeled and sliced
1 cup frozen peas
½ red bell pepper, seeded and diced
2 eggs, lightly beaten
Salt
3 tablespoons vegetable oil
1 small onion, finely chopped
1 scallion, finely sliced
1 to 2 tablespoons soy sauce

Wash the rice thoroughly and cook according to the package instructions in a saucepan of lightly salted water. Steam the carrot, peas, and red pepper until tender (about 5 minutes). Season the eggs with a little salt and fry them in a frying pan with 1 tablespoon of the oil until set as a thin omelet. Roll up into a sausage shape and cut into thin strips. Meanwhile, put the remaining 2 tablespoons oil into a wok or frying pan and sauté the chopped onion until softened. Add the rice and steamed vegetables and cook, stirring, for 2 to 3 minutes. Add the egg and scallion and cook, stirring, for 2 minutes more. Sprinkle with the soy sauce before serving.

Brown rice *tends not to be used for Chinese fried rice, but it is an excellent source of energy. It's a good idea to get your child used to eating brown rice, as it contains more minerals, vitamins, and fiber than white rice and is therefore much more nutritious.*

SUPERFOODS

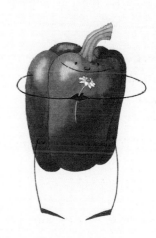

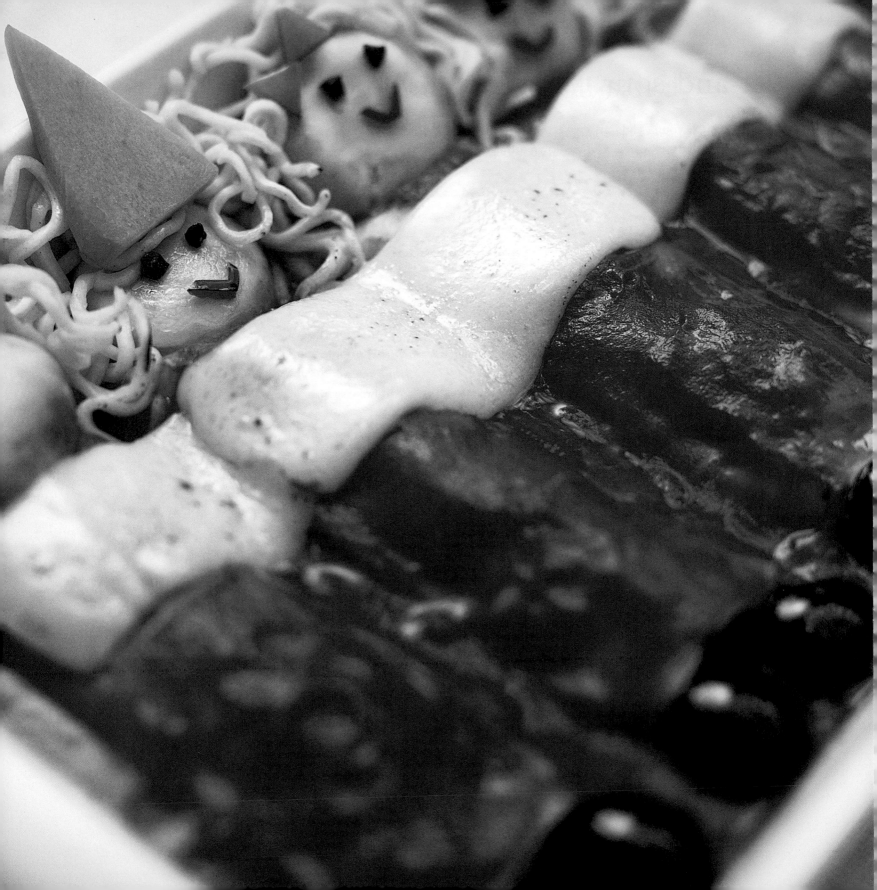

Spinach and ricotta cannelloni

 8 portions

This spinach filling is quick and easy to prepare, and there are some good-quality prepared tomato sauces available that can be used to cover the cannelloni if you haven't the time to make your own homemade sauce.

TOMATO SAUCE

1 medium onion, finely chopped

1 clove garlic, crushed

1 bay leaf

1 tablespoon olive oil

2 cups tomato puree

½ teaspoon sugar

Salt and freshly ground black pepper

One 10-ounce package frozen spinach, or 1 pound fresh

1 tablespoon butter

½ cup ricotta cheese

¼ cup grated Parmesan cheese

⅓ cup grated mozzarella cheese

Pinch of freshly grated nutmeg

Salt and freshly ground black pepper

8 no-boil cannelloni or lasagne sheets

Slices of Cheddar cheese

DECORATION

8 sautéed button mushrooms

20 pitted black olives

3 ounces cooked thin egg noodles

¼ red bell pepper, seeded

¼ green bell pepper, seeded

1 carrot, peeled

Preheat the oven to 350°F.

To make the tomato sauce, sauté the onion, garlic, and bay leaf in the olive oil for 2 minutes. Add the tomato puree and sugar, season to taste with salt and pepper, and simmer uncovered for about 8 minutes or until thickened. Remove the bay leaf from the tomato sauce.

Cook the spinach according to the package instructions. Drain well and press out any excess liquid with a wooden spoon, then roughly chop the spinach. Melt the butter in a saucepan and sauté the spinach for 1 to 2 minutes. Add the ricotta, Parmesan, and mozzarella cheeses and season to taste with nutmeg, salt, and pepper. Use this mixture to fill the cannelloni and arrange these in a single layer in a suitable ovenproof dish, leaving enough room for the mushroom faces and olive feet (see photograph). Cover with the tomato sauce. Bake for 25 to 30 minutes. Arrange the cheese slices over the tomato sauce to form a turned-down sheet and heat in the oven until melted.

To decorate, arrange the mushrooms as faces and add tiny triangles of black olive for eyes, thin egg noodles for hair with red and green pepper bows, carrot triangles for hats, and tiny strips of red pepper for the mouths. Finally, arrange the remaining black olives as feet.

Cheese *and dairy products contain calcium that can be absorbed by the body much more easily than calcium from other foods. Hard cheeses like Parmesan and Cheddar contain more calcium than soft cheeses like ricotta and cottage cheese. Eating cheese at the end of a meal can also help to fight tooth decay caused by sugary foods by reducing the acid levels in plaque, so the French tradition of finishing a meal with a little cheese is a good idea.*

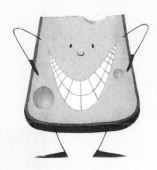

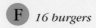

Chicken *provides a good source of high-value protein and all the essential amino acids that are so important for growing muscles. Chicken also contains the antioxidant selenium, which helps to protect us from heart disease and some cancers.*

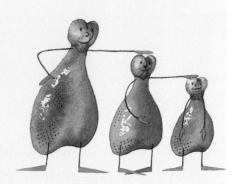

Delicious chicken burgers

Children love burgers and fast food. You can make your own healthy version using chicken and four different vegetables.

¼ cup washed and finely chopped white part of a leek
1 medium onion, finely chopped
2 medium carrots, peeled and grated
1 large zucchini, grated
1½ tablespoons vegetable oil
2 boneless, skinless chicken breasts, chopped
1 apple, peeled, cored, and grated
1 chicken stock cube, finely crumbled
1 tablespoon finely chopped fresh parsley
Salt and freshly ground black pepper
1½ cups bread crumbs

COATING
All-purpose flour
2 eggs, lightly beaten
Seasoned bread crumbs

Vegetable oil for frying

Sauté the leek, onion, carrots, and zucchini in the 1½ tablespoons vegetable oil for 3 minutes, then mix together with the remaining ingredients and chop in a food processor for a few seconds. Form into 16 burgers using floured hands.

Coat in flour, then egg, and then seasoned bread crumbs and sauté in vegetable oil until golden and cooked through (about 6 minutes on each side).

Beef in hoisin sauce with broccoli and water chestnuts

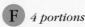

Marinating beef not only gives it a delicious flavor but also makes it more tender. I like to make this using round steak, which is a little cheaper than proper sirloin but still lovely and tender. Serve with noodles or rice.

MARINADE

2 tablespoons hoisin sauce

1 tablespoon soy sauce

1 tablespoon brown sugar

1 tablespoon sake (rice wine) or mirin

12 ounces tender beef, such as
   round steak, cut into strips

2½ tablespoons sunflower oil

1 clove garlic, crushed

1 medium onion, sliced

¼ cup sliced red or yellow bell pepper

2 cups small broccoli florets

1 cup sliced button mushrooms

One 8-ounce can sliced water chestnuts,
   drained

1 tablespoon cornstarch

1 cup beef stock

Mix together the marinade ingredients. Stir in the beef and leave to marinate for about 30 minutes. Heat 1 tablespoon of the oil in a wok and stir-fry half the garlic and onion for 3 minutes. Drain the beef, reserving the marinade, add the beef to the wok, and stir-fry for 4 minutes. Remove the beef and onion from the wok.

Clean the wok and heat the remaining 1½ tablespoons oil. Stir-fry the remaining onion and garlic for 3 minutes. Add the bell pepper and stir-fry for 2 minutes. Add the broccoli, mushrooms, and water chestnuts and stir-fry for 3 minutes.

Mix the cornstarch with 1 tablespoon water. Add to the vegetables in the wok together with the reserved marinade and the beef stock, and bring to a boil. Return the meat to the wok and simmer for 2 to 3 minutes.

Broccoli *is consistently associated with a lower risk of cancer if eaten regularly enough. It contains a variety of phytochemicals (biologically active non-nutrients), which can block cancer-causing agents before they reach their target sites or remove them before they cause damage. The American National Cancer Institute ranks it as the number one cancer-fighting vegetable. Scientists are trying genetically to inject these anticancer properties into other plants.*

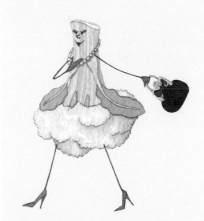

Singapore stir-fried noodles

SUPERFOODS

Shrimp *is rich in selenium and zinc, both of which are important to maintaining a strong immune system. Zinc is also important for repair and healing. The noodles are a good source of carbohydrates for energy.*

Warning: *Always be sure that shellfish is fresh. Shellfish past its prime is a common cause of food poisoning.*

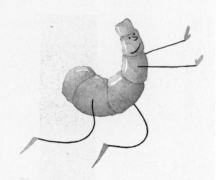

Offering foods from around the world will broaden your child's tastes, and this dish should prove to be popular with the whole family. Too many children have a boring and repetitive diet of hamburgers, fries, pizza, and other stereotyped "children's foods." There are now so many other choices available to us, especially with the greater variety of international foods available in supermarkets like rice noodles, fresh ginger, and korma curry paste. Don't be afraid to make some more exotic dishes for your children—their tastes are often more sophisticated than we give them credit for.

6 ounces rice noodles or fine Chinese egg noodles
1 tablespoon vegetable oil
1/2 clove garlic, crushed
1/4 green chile, finely diced
1/4 teaspoon finely grated gingerroot
1 small boneless, skinless chicken breast, cut into very small pieces
2/3 cup frozen peas
2 ounces cooked small shrimp, peeled
2 scallions, finely sliced
1 tablespoon soy sauce
1 tablespoon sake (rice wine) or mirin
Pinch of sugar
2 teaspoons mild korma curry paste
1/2 cup chicken stock
1 egg, lightly beaten
Salt and white pepper

Place the rice noodles in a large bowl and cover with boiling water. Leave to stand for 3 minutes. If using Chinese noodles, follow the cooking instructions on the package. Drain in a colander and then rinse thoroughly in cold water and leave to drain. Heat the oil in a wok and sauté the garlic, chile, and gingerroot for 1 minute. Add the chicken and stir-fry for 2 minutes. Add the peas, shrimp, and scallions. Add the noodles and soy sauce, rice wine, sugar, curry paste, and stock. Add the lightly beaten egg and cook, stirring, for 1 to 2 minutes. Season to taste with salt and pepper.

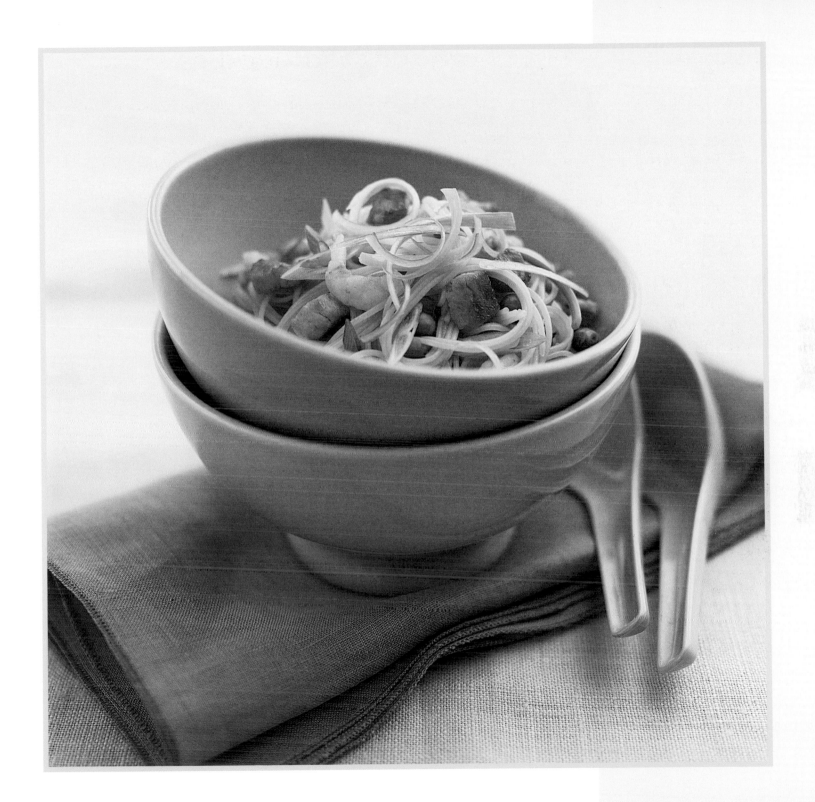

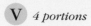

Cheesy baked potato with butternut squash

4 medium baking potatoes
  (approximately 8 ounces each)
Vegetable oil
½ medium butternut squash (10 ounces)
3 tablespoons butter plus a little extra

1 teaspoon Dijon mustard
⅓ cup grated Parmesan cheese
2 tablespoons milk
Salt and freshly ground black pepper
½ cup grated Cheddar cheese

Preheat the oven to 375°F. Prick the potatoes in several places, place on a baking sheet, and brush all over with oil. Bake for 1 to 1½ hours or until they feel soft when pressed. Meanwhile, scoop out the seeds from the squash half and brush the flesh with a little soft butter. Bake in the oven for 45 to 50 minutes or until tender. When cool enough to handle, cut the tops off the potatoes and scoop out the flesh. Scoop the flesh from the cooked squash and mash together with the potato, the mustard, Parmesan, milk, and butter. Season to taste with salt and pepper. Put the mixture back into the potato shells, top with the grated Cheddar, and place under the broiler for a few minutes until golden.

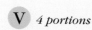

Vegetable tempura and dipping sauce

Vegetable oil for frying

TEMPURA BATTER
¾ cup all-purpose flour
½ cup cornstarch
1 cup ice-cold carbonated water
  (add 2 ice cubes if necessary)

Selection of vegetables, such as zucchini,
  carrot, sweet potato, broccoli, and
cauliflower
Coarse sea salt

DIPPING SAUCE
¼ cup rice wine vinegar
1 tablespoon light brown sugar
1 teaspoon grated gingerroot (optional)
¼ cup sake (rice wine) or mirin
1 tablespoon soy sauce
1 red chile, seeded and finely sliced
1 tablespoon finely sliced scallion

Preheat a deep-fat fryer to 375°F or heat about 3 inches of the oil in a wok or frying pan. To check if the oil is at the correct temperature, drop a small cube of bread into the oil. If the bread sizzles and turns crisp and golden, the oil is ready to use.

While the oil is heating, put the flour and cornstarch in a large bowl and then with the handle of a wooden spoon, mix and stir in the ice-cold water until the mixture takes on the consistency of heavy cream. Only mix very lightly, as it should be quite lumpy.

Cut the zucchini into batons, the carrot and sweet potato into thin strips, and the broccoli and cauliflower into florets. Dip the vegetables in the batter. Deep-fry a few vegetables at a time; don't crowd the deep-fat fryer with too many vegetables, or you will bring down the temperature of the oil. When the batter turns golden, remove the vegetables from the pan using a slotted spoon and drain on paper towels. Season with a good sprinkling of sea salt.

To make the sauce, put the vinegar and sugar in a pan, bring to a boil, and then simmer for 3 minutes or until slightly reduced. (If using gingerroot, add to the pan in the last minute of cooking.) Add the rice wine and bring to a boil, then remove from the heat and stir in the soy sauce. Allow to cool a little, and then stir in the chile and scallion.

Cheat's cheese soufflé

This comes out of the oven all puffed up with a lovely golden cheese crust, so it's a bit like a wholesome cheese soufflé, and just like a soufflé, it's best eaten right away.

2 tablespoons butter, plus extra
   for greasing
3 medium onions, finely sliced
1 teaspoon chopped fresh thyme
1 clove garlic, crushed
Salt and freshly ground black pepper
½ cup grated Parmesan cheese

½ cup grated Cheddar cheese
½ cup grated Swiss cheese
8 to 10 slices white bread, crusts removed
3 large eggs
2 cups whole milk
½ teaspoon mustard powder,
   such as Colman's

Preheat the oven to 375°F. Melt the butter in a large saucepan and gently sauté the onions until softened and lightly golden (about 10 minutes). Stir in the thyme and garlic and season with salt and pepper; allow to cool slightly. Combine the cheeses and stir into the onions.

Butter an ovenproof dish and lay in half of the bread and then sprinkle with half of the cheese and onion mixture. Top with the remaining bread and sprinkle with the remaining cheese and onion. Mix together the eggs, milk, and mustard powder and season with salt and pepper. Pour this over the cheese and bread and leave to soak for about 10 minutes. Bake for 25 to 30 minutes.

 V *8 portions*

Whole-grain bread

is an excellent source of complex carbohydrates for energy and fiber as well as of vitamins and minerals. Although white and brown bread don't contain all the fiber and natural goodness, they are still nutritious, particularly as they are fortified with iron, calcium, nicotinic acid, and vitamin B_1. Bread is also a good source of carbohydrates, which are used as energy.

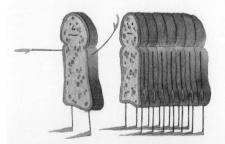

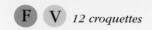

Potatoes *provide us with a good source of complex carbohydrates, which are a good source of energy. They also contain vitamin C, potassium, and—as long as they remain unpeeled—fiber. Baked potatoes are very good for children, and you can top them with baked beans for added fiber.*

Vegetable croquettes

These tasty vegetable croquettes are made with mashed potato, broccoli, and grated carrot, are flavored with Swiss cheese, and have a crispy golden bread crumb coating.

2 medium potatoes, peeled
1½ cups small broccoli florets
1 medium onion, chopped
1 clove garlic, crushed
1 tablespoon butter
½ cup grated carrot
1 cup grated Swiss cheese

Salt and freshly ground pepper
All-purpose flour seasoned with salt
   and pepper
2 eggs, lightly beaten
1½ cups bread crumbs
Vegetable oil for sautéing

Cook the potatoes in a large pot of lightly salted boiling water for 20 minutes. Steam the broccoli for 4 minutes. Chop the broccoli into small pieces. Sauté the onion and garlic in the butter for 2 minutes, add the carrot, and sauté for 1 minute. Drain and mash the potatoes and mix in the cheese. Then mix in the broccoli, onion, and carrot. Season with salt and pepper.

Form into burgers. Coat with seasoned flour, dip in the beaten egg, then the bread crumbs, then the egg, and then give a final coating of bread crumbs. Sauté in vegetable oil until golden.

4 portions

Pasta *is a good source of carbohydrates. It is also a good source of B vitamins and complex carbohydrates that will keep young bodies going for hours.*

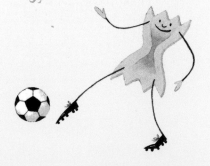

Bow-tie pasta salad with tuna

6 ounces bow-tie pasta
1 shallot, very finely chopped
One 6-ounce can tuna in oil,
   drained and flaked
4 cherry tomatoes, quartered
⅔ cup cooked frozen or canned corn
1 small avocado, peeled, pitted,
   and cut into small cubes

DRESSING
2 tablespoons mayonnaise
2 tablespoons olive oil
2 teaspoons lemon juice
Pinch of cayenne pepper

Cook the pasta according to the package instructions.

In a bowl, mix together all the remaining ingredients for the salad, but don't add the avocado until just before serving, or it will discolor. Mix together the ingredients for the dressing. Drain the pasta, and when cool, mix with the salad and toss in the dressing.

Salmon teriyaki with noodles

It's easy to make your own delicious teriyaki sauce.

MARINADE

2 tablespoons rice wine vinegar

2 tablespoons dark brown sugar

2 tablespoons soy sauce

1 tablespoon Asian sesame oil

10 ounces salmon, cut into small cubes

1 tablespoon vegetable oil

1 clove garlic, crushed

¼ teaspoon grated gingerroot

4 small scallions, thinly sliced

1 cup bean sprouts

1 cup sugar snap peas

1 tablespoon cornstarch

¼ cup fish stock or water

6 ounces thin egg noodles

Mix together the ingredients for the marinade and marinate the salmon for about 30 minutes. Remove the salmon with a slotted spoon and reserve the marinade. Heat the vegetable oil in a pan and stir-fry the salmon with the garlic and gingerroot until opaque on the outside (about 1 minute). Remove with a slotted spoon. Stir-fry the scallions, bean sprouts, and sugar snap peas for 1 minute.

Mix the cornstarch into 1 tablespoon of the reserved marinade and add to the pan together with the remaining marinade and the stock or water. Bring the mixture to a boil and simmer until thickened (about 1 minute). Cook the noodles according to the package instructions and drain. Add the noodles and salmon to the vegetables in the pan and heat through for about 1 minute.

4 portions

Oily fish *such as salmon is one of the few nutritional sources of the omega-3 polyunsaturated fatty acids that are essential for good health and have many health-giving properties. Fish fats are polyunsaturated fats, which means they flow rather than being solid like butter. These liquid-type fats are important to prevent the clogging of arteries, which is important in the prevention of heart disease and strokes in adults. Interestingly, the Inuit people, whose diet is high in fish oils, do not have a high incidence of heart disease—possibly because they consume large amounts of the right type of fat.*

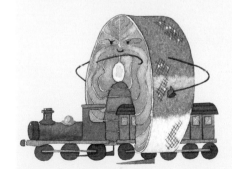

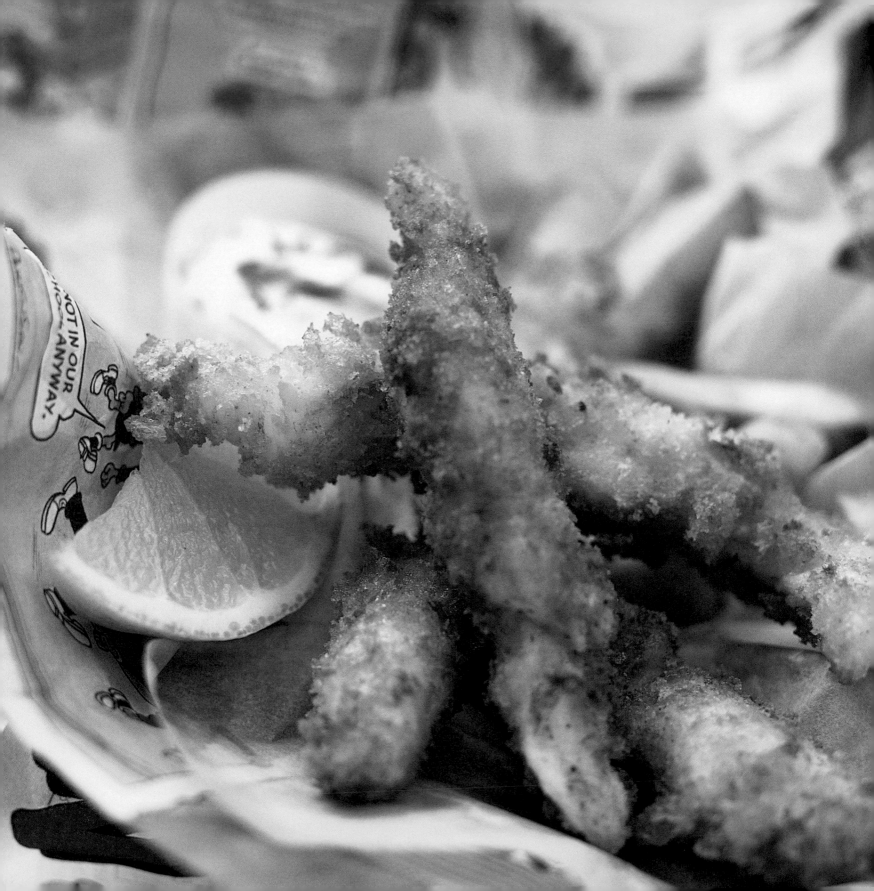

Fish and chips in a comic

3 portions

Serve these strips of fish with french fries—and how about wrapping them in a comic book instead of a newspaper for added child appeal? If you wish, you can line the comic with some waxed paper.

Sunflower oil for frying
5 ounces sole or flounder fillet, skinned
¼ cup all-purpose flour
Salt and freshly ground black pepper
Cayenne pepper
1 egg, lightly beaten
1¼ cups bread crumbs

TARTAR SAUCE
½ cup mayonnaise
Lemon juice to taste
1 tablespoon chopped fresh parsley
1½ tablespoons chopped capers
2 teaspoons chopped gherkins
1 tablespoon snipped chives

Preheat a deep-fryer to 375°F or heat about 3 inches of the oil in a wok or frying pan.

Cut the fish into strips and coat in flour seasoned with salt and pepper and cayenne pepper. Dip the coated fish into the egg and then coat the strips in the bread crumbs and deep-fry for 3 to 4 minutes in two batches.

To make the tartar sauce, simply mix together all the ingredients and serve with the fish and chips.

Fish *is a nutrient-dense source of protein and also a good source of vitamin B_{12}. It is a good idea to include fish dishes regularly to allow children to get used to this very useful and healthy food in our diets.*

SUPERFOODS

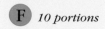 *10 portions*

Tuna *is a true SuperFood pantry standby, rich in protein, vitamin D, and vitamin B$_{12}$. Tuna is rich in omega-3 fatty acids, which help to protect us against heart disease.*

Tuna tagliatelle

This is both a tasty and nutritious pasta dish. To make things easier you can sometimes cheat a little and combine convenience foods with fresh foods. Here I have used a can of cream of tomato soup and a can of tuna, which are handy pantry ingredients.

TOMATO AND TUNA SAUCE
½ medium onion, finely chopped
2 tablespoons butter, plus extra
   for greasing pan
1 tablespoon cornstarch
One 10.75-ounce can cream of tomato soup
Pinch of mixed dried herbs,
   such as Italian Seasoning
1 tablespoon chopped fresh parsley
One 6-ounce can tuna in olive oil,
   drained and flaked
Freshly ground black pepper

MUSHROOM CHEESE SAUCE
½ medium onion, finely chopped
3 tablespoons butter
1 cup sliced button mushrooms
2 tablespoons all-purpose flour
1¼ cups whole milk
1 cup grated Cheddar cheese

6 ounces green tagliatelle
1 tablespoon grated Parmesan cheese

To make the tomato and tuna sauce, sauté the onion in the butter in a pan until soft. Stir the cornstarch into ½ cup water until dissolved, and mix with the tomato soup. Add to the pan along with the mixed herbs and chopped parsley and cook, stirring, over low heat for 5 minutes. Mix in the tuna and heat through. Season with a little pepper.

For the mushroom cheese sauce, sauté the onion in the butter until transparent, then add the mushrooms and sauté for about 3 minutes. Add the flour, stirring constantly. When it is well mixed, add the milk gradually and cook, stirring, until thickened and smooth. Remove from the heat and stir in the cheese.

Preheat the oven to 350°F. Cook the tagliatelle in a large pot of lightly salted boiling water until al dente and then drain. Mix the tagliatelle with the tuna and tomato sauce. Grease a lasagne dish that measures about 8 inches square and spoon half the tuna and tomato tagliatelle into the dish. Top with half the mushroom cheese sauce. Spoon in the remaining tuna and tomato tagliatelle and top with the rest of the mushroom cheese sauce. Finish off by sprinkling the Parmesan cheese on top. Bake for 20 minutes and brown under a hot broiler before serving.

Bow-tie pasta with salmon and tomatoes

Combining pasta with less popular foods like fish is a good way to encourage children to eat them. This tasty recipe takes only a few minutes to prepare.

6 ounces bow-tie pasta
7 ounces salmon fillet, skinned
1 pat butter
Salt and freshly ground black pepper
6 tablespoons sour cream
½ cup ketchup
1 tablespoon snipped chives
3 plum tomatoes, peeled, seeded, and chopped

Cook the pasta in a large pot of lightly salted boiling water according to the instructions on the package. Put the salmon into a suitable microwave dish, dot with the butter, and season with salt and pepper. Cover with microwave-safe plastic wrap, pierce a few times, and cook for 2 to 2½ minutes, according to the thickness of the fish. Strain and reserve the juices from the fish.

Heat the sour cream, ketchup, and fish juices in a large pan, stirring until blended. Add the chives and tomatoes, season to taste with salt and pepper, and simmer for 1 minute. Carefully flake the salmon, checking that there are no bones, and add to the sauce. Drain the pasta and toss with the sauce.

4 portions

Salmon *is good for the heart. Eating oily fish like salmon can help protect against heart attacks and strokes by helping to keep blood flowing freely, thus reducing the risk of a blood clot forming within a blood vessel. The darker the fish, the higher the levels of fat, so make sure that you include some dark fish in your child's diet at least once or twice a week.*

SUPERFOODS

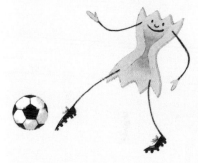

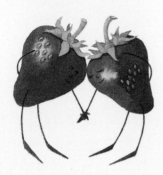
Strawberry and rhubarb crumble

This is a delicious combination of flavors, and the pink color of the rhubarb looks so attractive. It is also quick and easy to prepare. Serve with custard sauce or ice cream.

TOPPING

1 cup all-purpose flour

Salt

8 tablespoons (1 stick) cold butter, cut into pieces

1/2 cup light brown sugar

1/2 cup ground almonds

FILLING

1 1/2 tablespoons ground almonds

1 pound rhubarb, cut into small pieces

6 hulled and halved strawberries

1/4 cup superfine sugar

Preheat the oven to 400°F. To make the topping, mix the flour together with a generous pinch of salt in a bowl and rub in the butter using your fingertips until the mixture resembles bread crumbs. Then rub in the brown sugar and ground almonds.

For the filling, sprinkle the ground almonds over the base of a suitable ovenproof dish (a round Pyrex dish 8 inches in diameter is good). Mix the rhubarb and strawberries together with the sugar, and spoon into the dish. Cover the fruit with the crumble topping and sprinkle with 1 tablespoon of water, which will help to make the topping crispy. Bake until the topping becomes a golden brown (about 25 minutes).

Fruity gelatin

You can add any fruit to Jell-O except fresh pineapple, kiwifruit, or papaya; they will prevent it from jelling. You can also make this in a bowl instead of molds.

One 3-ounce package peach, strawberry, or raspberry gelatin dessert mix

1 orange, peeled, cut into segments, and pith removed

1/2 cup halved seedless black or red grapes

1/2 cup raspberries or blueberries

6 hulled and quartered strawberries

1 peach, peeled, pitted, and cut into pieces, or use canned peaches in juice

Make the gelatin according to the package instructions and set aside to cool. Divide the fruits among four 7-ounce individual molds, then pour in the gelatin. Chill in the refrigerator until set. Dip the molds in hot water and turn out.

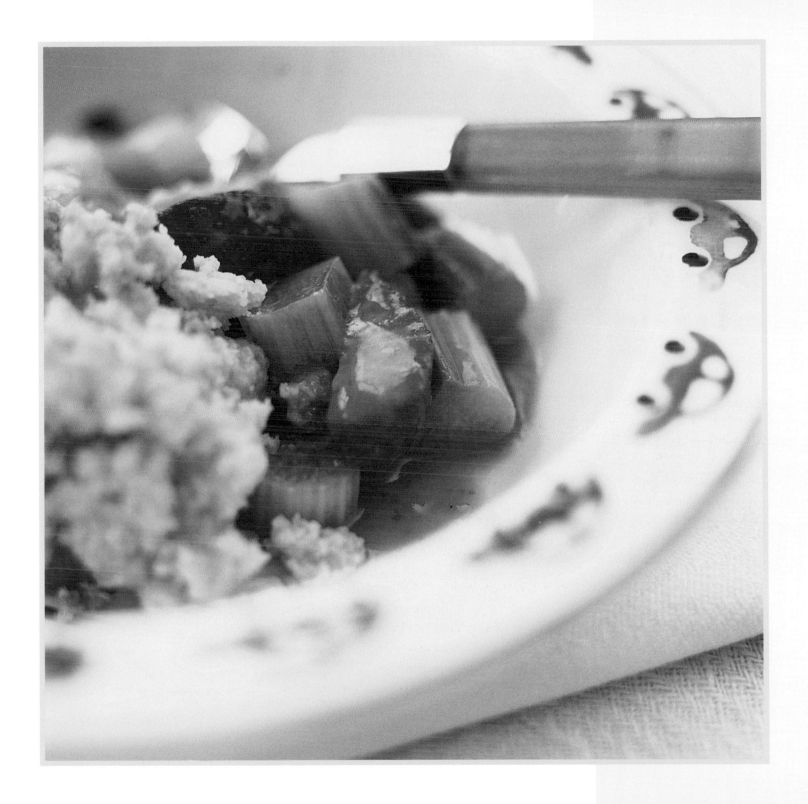

Chocolate *increases levels of serotonin in the brain, which helps lift your mood. Good-quality dark chocolate is a rich source of iron and magnesium, which are essential to bone health.*

Good news for chocolate lovers! Research published by the British Medical Journal *suggests that a daily meal of seven ingredients (which includes 3½ ounces of dark chocolate along with fish, fruit, vegetables, almonds, garlic, and wine) could cut the risk of coronary heart disease by a massive 76 percent. Scientists predict this could increase average life expectancy by six years. Eating 3½ ounces of dark chocolate per day could reduce blood pressure and reduce the risk of heart attack or stroke by 21 percent.*

Lara's favorite brownies

These are absolutely delicious; I find that children prefer brownies without walnut pieces. My daughter Lara is sixteen and adores chocolate, and she loves to make these brownies and share them with her friends. They are great served with a scoop of vanilla ice cream and hot chocolate sauce. (Good news for teenagers: the fear that chocolate can cause acne is not supported by any scientific evidence.)

1½ sticks unsalted butter, plus extra for greasing
4½ ounces good-quality bittersweet chocolate, broken into pieces
3 large eggs
¾ cup light brown sugar or superfine sugar
¾ cup ground almonds
⅔ cup all-purpose flour
⅓ cup chocolate chips
⅓ cup chopped white chocolate
Confectioners' sugar for dusting

Preheat the oven to 350°F. Cut the butter into pieces and put into a heatproof bowl together with the bittersweet chocolate. Place the bowl over a pan of simmering water and stir until melted. Beat the eggs and sugar together with an electric mixer for about 5 minutes or until thickened and fluffy. Stir in the melted chocolate mixture. Fold in the ground almonds, flour, chocolate chips, and white chocolate.

Grease and line an 8-inch square cake pan and pour the mixture into the pan. Bake for about 30 minutes or until well risen and slightly firm at the edges. The brownies will still be soft in the center. Leave to cool in the pan, then turn out and dust the top with sifted confectioners' sugar. Cut into squares before serving.

Fruit smoothies

Peach passions

For variety, add two strawberries or substitute strawberries for the peach.

Juice of 1 large orange
1 large juicy peach, peeled, pitted, and cut into pieces
½ small banana

Simply blend together all the ingredients.

Tropical treat

You could also make this using peach instead of banana. Choose passion fruit with wrinkly skins, as this shows the fruit is ripe.

1 cup chopped mango flesh
1 small or ½ medium banana
Juice of 1 orange
1 passion fruit (optional)
Honey, to taste

Blend together the mango, banana, and orange juice. If using, cut the passion fruit in half. Scoop out the pulp and stir in, adding a little honey to taste.

Nectarine and strawberry

Frozen bananas make wonderful smoothies. Pop a banana in the freezer, unpeeled, for about 3 hours.

1 small frozen banana
2 large juicy nectarines or peaches, peeled, pitted, and cut into pieces

4 strawberries, hulled and cut in half
½ cup orange juice
¾ cup vanilla yogurt

Cut the banana into chunks. Puree all the ingredients in a blender until smooth.

 1 large or 2 small smoothies

Smoothies *are good for breakfast or a snack. They are naturally high in antioxidants because they are made with fresh fruit.*

Healthy eating:
If you are struggling to get your child to eat the recommended five portions of fruit and vegetables per day, try making fruit smoothies using fresh and canned fruit. Any fruits can be used. Allow older children to join in by cutting and peeling the fruits. They can also experiment with different flavors. Ice cream can be added to sweeten if needed.

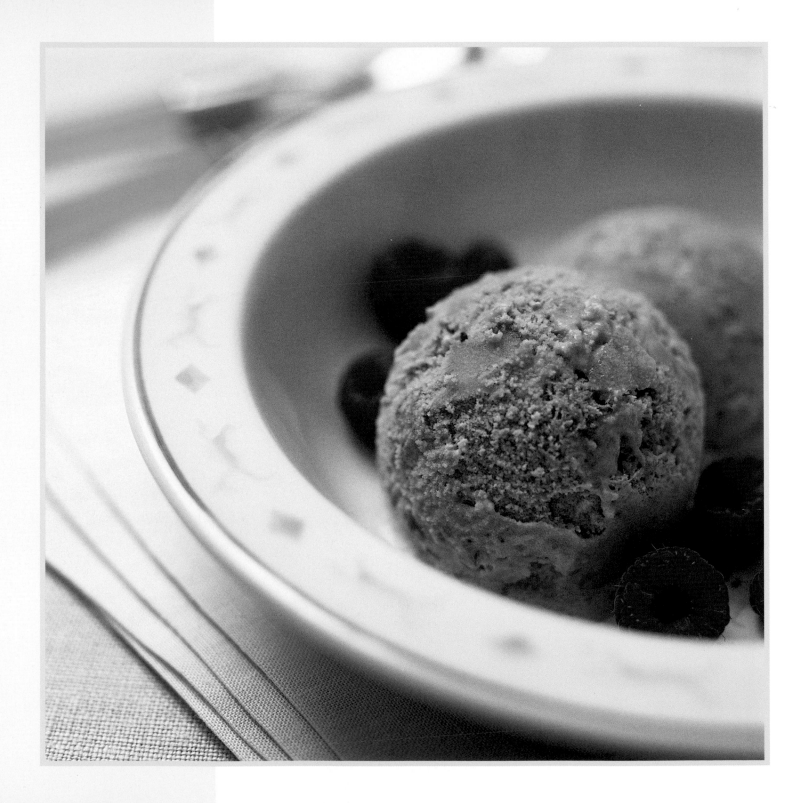

Peach melba frozen yogurt with crushed meringues

A new twist to the classic peach melba—children will love the crunchy pieces of meringue in this frozen yogurt.

8 ounces fresh raspberries
Two 15-ounce cans peach halves, drained
2 cups (16 ounces) plain yogurt
½ cup sifted confectioners' sugar
1 cup heavy cream
3 ounces crumbled meringues or vanilla wafers

Puree the raspberries and puree three-quarters of the peaches. Chop the rest and set aside. Mix together the yogurt, sugar, and pureed fruits. Add the cream and blend in a food processor for about 30 seconds. Freeze in an ice cream–making machine, and toward the end of the freezing time stir in the reserved peaches and the meringues. Alternatively, put into a suitable container and freeze for 1½ hours, remove from the freezer, add the reserved peaches and the meringues, and stir thoroughly. Freeze for another hour and stir again.

8 portions

Live yogurt *contains good bacteria that maintain the balance of good and bad bacteria in our guts and can help prevent illness. If a child develops diarrhea on antibiotics, it may be a good idea to give her live yogurt. Antibiotics kill off bad and good bacteria in the intestine and eating live yogurt helps to restore the balance.*

Fruit-flavored yogurts may claim to be low in fat but may contain large amounts of sugar or artificial sweetener.

Healthy eating:

There is a lot of hype about good bacteria added to yogurts and drinks, as it may help prevent the overgrowth of bad "bugs" in our large intestines. But many "live" yogurts contain bacteria that don't make it past the acid in our stomachs. Check that the yogurt contains lactobacillus or bifidobacterium.

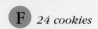

Raisins *are a concentrated source of calories and fiber and provide a high-energy snack. They are good mixed with oats for these cookies, since the high sugar content of raisins provides a quick release of energy while the oats provide sustained energy. Raisins are also a source of iron.*

Chewy oatmeal raisin cookies

These delicious cookies are quick and easy to make and very more-ish. If you like, you can add a little ground cinnamon to flavor them.

1 stick unsalted butter, plus extra for greasing	1 cup all-purpose flour
1 cup superfine sugar	1 teaspoon baking powder
1 cup light brown sugar	½ teaspoon salt
1 egg	1 cup rolled oats
1 teaspoon pure vanilla extract	¾ cup raisins

Preheat the oven to 350°F. Beat the butter together with the sugars until light and fluffy. Beat in the egg and vanilla. Combine the flour, baking powder, salt, and oats and stir this into the creamed butter and sugar mixture. Finally, stir in the raisins.

Prepare two large greased or lined baking sheets. Form the mixture into walnut-size balls and flatten them with your fingers onto the baking sheets. Space them well apart. Bake for about 15 minutes or until the edges are a light golden brown.

Kiwifruit *contains almost twice as much vitamin C as oranges. One kiwifruit supplies more than the daily adult requirement of vitamin C. The dark color of the flesh means it is packed full of goodness.*

Traffic light ice pops

No child can resist an ice pop. Unfortunately, most store-bought pops are full of sugar and artificial colorings and flavorings. If peaches are not in season, you could use fresh orange juice. It's easy to make your own pops by simply pouring fruit juice or smoothies into ice pop molds or small yogurt containers.

6 large strawberries	3 large juicy peaches or nectarines, peeled, pitted, and sliced
4½ tablespoons honey	5 large kiwifruit, peeled and sliced

In a blender, puree the strawberries and then strain. Stir 1½ tablespoons of the honey into the strawberry puree. Then pour the strawberry puree into each of the ice pop molds until each mold is one-third full, and freeze until firm (about 1½ hours). Repeat this process with the peaches and 1½ tablespoons of the honey (no need to strain peaches), and then puree the kiwifruit (strain the puree) and mix with the remaining 1½ tablespoons honey.

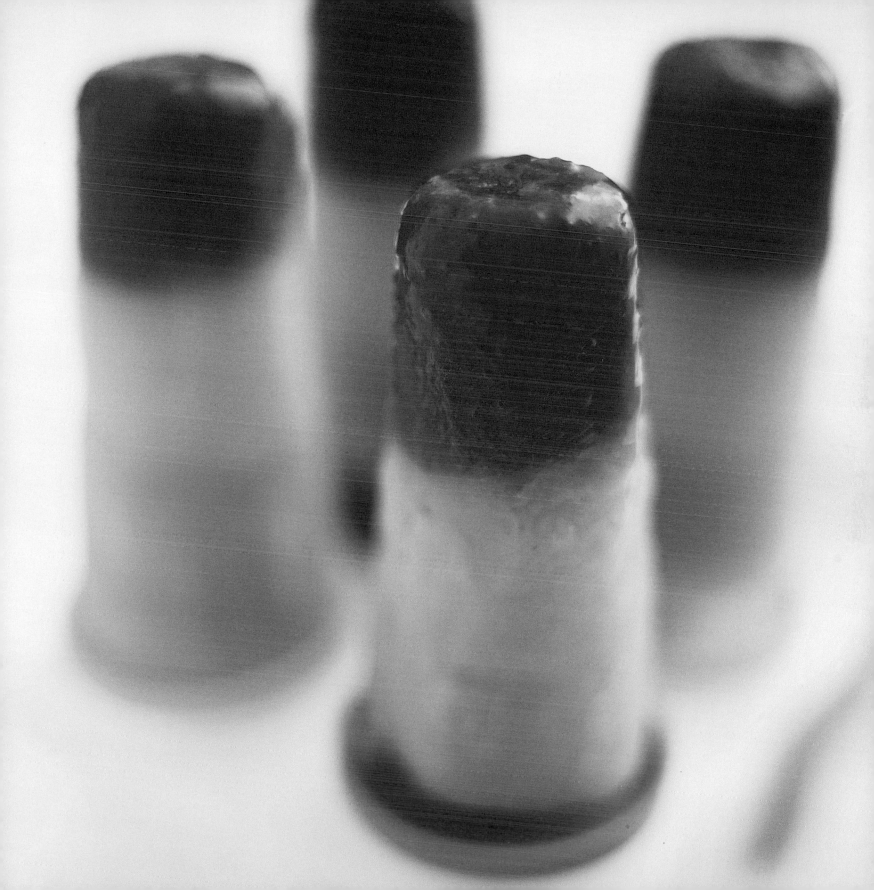

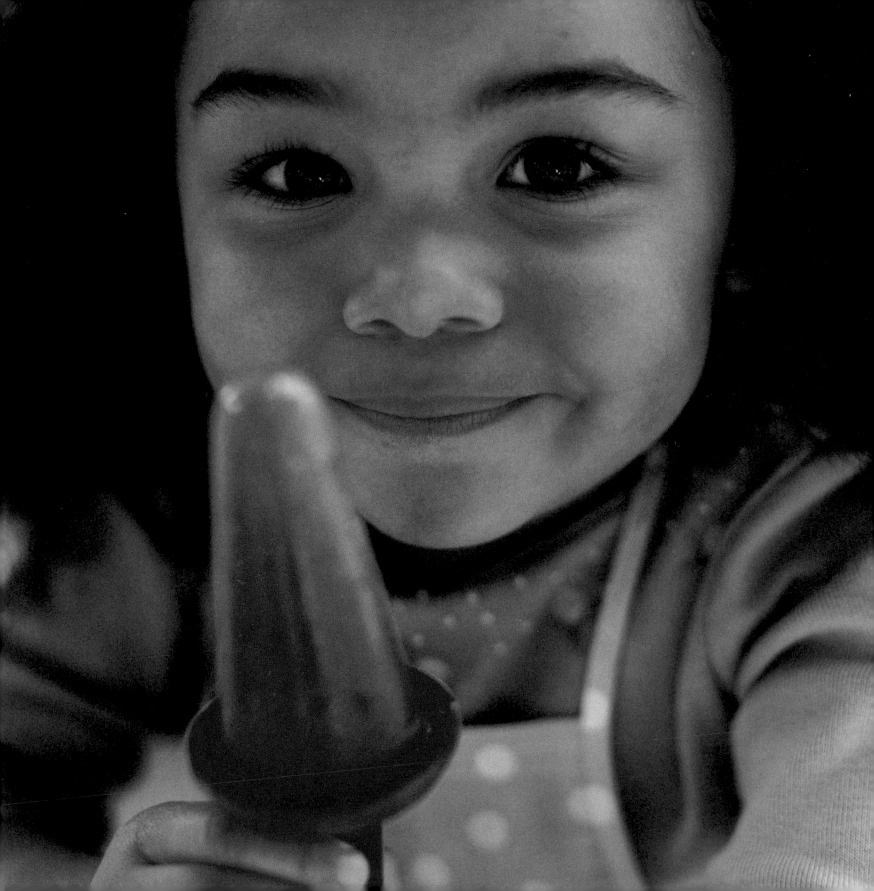

3 years plus:

favorite family meals

To make food a fun and enjoyable experience for your child, involve her in shopping and cooking. Encourage her to be adventurous and to try some of the wonderful dishes from around the world in this chapter.

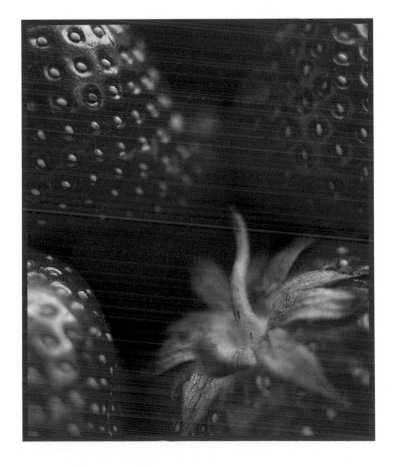

Favorite family meals

Between the ages of three and five, your child's manual dexterity should improve and she should master eating with a knife and fork. She should have her first full set of teeth. Nearly all the recipes in this section are designed as family meals but include that magical ingredient of child appeal.

The big change in your child's life at this stage will probably be starting preschool. Eating has to fit more into a routine. Young children will need a good breakfast to keep them alert until lunchtime. You may also need to make a packed lunch for school, which should be both appealing and nutritious.

Young children are more likely to accept new tastes than older children, so it is important to introduce as much variety as possible at a young age. A lot of my inspiration for writing recipe books for children comes from looking at foods from around the world and then finding ways to make them child-friendly as well as quick and easy to prepare for busy parents. I have found with my three children that they adore Chinese, Indian, and Thai food—try my recipes for Chinese Fried Rice (page 123), Nasi Goreng (page 155), Thai-Style Chicken and Noodles (page 159), and Mild Beef Curry (page 167).

Is your child eating properly?

I know many mothers who constantly worry that their child is not eating enough, so how do you tell if a young child is getting all the nutrients he needs? If your child is growing properly, has plenty of energy, and seems healthy and strong, then even if he doesn't have an enormous appetite, he is probably absolutely fine. It is reassuring to know that toddlers can thrive on remarkably little food. They tend to be quite unpredictable and one day can be ravenous and the next have no appetite at all. It's much better to review a child's food intake over a period of a week rather than worrying on a day-to-day basis. If your child doesn't seem to be thriving, often gets ill, and seems listless, it is possible that he is not getting enough iron in his diet. Cow's milk, unlike formula milk, is a very poor source of iron and you will need to include some iron-rich foods like red meat, whole grains, dark green leafy vegetables, and lentils in his diet. Vitamin C enhances the body's absorption of iron, so give a vitamin C–rich fruit juice like orange or cranberry juice (¼ cup will do) with your child's meal.

The creative lunch box

Have you ever wondered why schoolchildren's learning, attention span, and behavior tend to deteriorate after lunch? The answer lies hidden in their lunch box. A recent survey found that an average lunch box contains potato chips and a chocolate bar, and very few children bring fresh fruit. A high-fat, high-salt, refined-carbohydrate meal such as this will leave your child feeling tired and unable to concentrate. Moreover, a diet high in saturated fat and salt can lay the foundations for heart disease and high blood pressure later in life.

A healthy lunch box should contain a balance of complex carbohydrates and protein, together with some fresh fruit and a drink. Your child's attention, behavior, and learning in the afternoon should then be just fine.

Making the lunch box more appetizing

When your child brings his lunch to school, he carries a little piece of home with him. When my three children each had to take a lunch box, it became a challenge to come up with something new to entice them to eat healthy food and bring a smile to their faces

Do children need vitamin supplements?

Vitamin pills are no substitute for fresh food. We are foolish if we think that we can beat nature at its own game. Man-made supplements can never hope to replace all the nutrients contained in food. Many of the phytonutrients that we now realize are important in beating cancer were thought of as poisonous some years ago. There may be other factors locked up in fresh produce that we are still unaware of. The point to remember is that supplements do not replace food, and a good diet will provide your child with all the vitamins and minerals she needs.

after a long morning at school. Simple touches can make all the difference, like drawing a face on your child's banana with a felt-tip pen and decorating it with stickers or cutting sandwiches into shapes using cookie cutters.

You can control what goes into your child's lunch box, but you can't control what goes into your child. I know it may seem obvious, but make sure you send your child to school with food in his lunch box that he likes. It is often a good idea, time permitting, to let your child get involved helping to pack his own lunch box or perhaps discuss with him the night before what he would like to include the following day.

Your child will probably only eat food in the school cafeteria that he feels comfortable eating. Most children are greatly influenced by peer pressure, and just because your child likes eating raw cauliflower with a dip at home doesn't mean he will be comfortable eating this sort of food at school. So you have to find foods that suit your nutritional standards and that are also acceptable among his social set.

Most children will leave food that takes a lot of effort to eat, as they want a quick refueling stop leaving maximum time for the playground. For example, give clementines already peeled or cut kiwifruit in half and let them scoop out the flesh with a teaspoon.

If your child likes potato chips but you don't want him to fill himself up by eating a whole bag, put some in a sealable plastic bag or wrap some in foil.

Something hot for winter

As the colder weather sets in it is a good idea to include something hot in a lunch box. A widemouthed mini thermos would be ideal for serving up a delicious cup of homemade or good-quality store-bought soup, which is both warming and nutritious—the perfect way to keep your child warm during lunchtime play.

Something cool for summer

Warm conditions encourage the growth of bacteria, so it is very important to keep lunch boxes cool. For the summer get a lunch box with a built-in ice pack to keep food fresh. Alternatively, put an individual carton of juice in the freezer overnight and transfer it to your child's lunch box in the morning, and by lunchtime it will have thawed and will have helped keep the food fresh.

Sandwiches

Sandwiches don't need to be boring. Presentation is very important to children. Vary the types of bread you use to make sandwiches. Try bagels or French, Italian, or raisin bread. Bread doesn't always need to be buttered, especially if you use ingredients like cream cheese or peanut butter. Wrap sandwiches in plastic wrap or aluminum foil or pack them in small plastic containers to prevent them from getting squashed. Here are some quick ways to turn an ordinary sandwich into something special.

Novelty-shaped sandwiches: Use a variety of cutters to shape sandwiches into animals, people, or cars. Popular fillings are peanut butter, cream cheese and cucumber, and egg salad and shredded lettuce. Peanut butter is always a popular filling and it can be used on its own or can go together with sliced or mashed banana, jelly, honey, or raisins.

Mini pita pockets: These make a welcome change. Possible fillings are flaked tuna with corn or sliced turkey with Swiss cheese and lettuce.

Mismatched sandwiches: You can encourage your child to eat whole-wheat bread by making sandwiches from one slice of whole-wheat and one slice of white bread. Cut them into quarters and pack with the alternate triangles uppermost.

Tortilla roll-ups: Make a change by giving your child food wrapped in a parcel like the Delicious Chicken Fajitas (page 164) or Tuna Tortilla Roll-ups (page 170). Flour tortillas are perfect for savory fillings.

Popular sandwich fillings

- Egg, tuna, or chicken salad with salad greens or watercress.
- Cream cheese and cucumber.
- Peanut butter and banana or whole fruit spreads.
- Bacon, lettuce, and tomato (with turkey bacon).
- Sliced turkey or ham with cheese.
- Grilled chicken breast with avocado and tomato.
- Ham, Swiss cheese, and cucumber.
- Hummus with grated carrot or cucumber.
- Shredded cheese with tomato and cucumber.
- Shrimp in cocktail sauce with shredded lettuce.
- Grated carrots and raisins with mayonnaise.
- Ham and sweet relish.

Kids in the kitchen

Children enjoy helping in the kitchen and are often more willing to eat foods that they have helped to prepare. However, cooking is sadly a vital missing ingredient from the school curriculum. Learning to cook is a basic survival skill. School may take care of reading, writing, and arithmetic, but if no one teaches children to cook, then it's likely that they will grow up reliant on processed, packaged foods.

Many five-year-olds are proficient at playing the latest computer games, but I wonder how many can squeeze orange juice or crack an egg. Children love to cook and relish tactile experiences like kneading and rolling out dough or breaking eggs, but the trouble is we very often don't allow them in the kitchen for fear of the mess. Children delight in the very ordinary tasks that we adults take for granted and managing these tasks gives them a wonderful sense of sharing and achievement.

On weekends, when there is more time, you can get your child involved in cooking breakfast. It's interesting how very often being involved in the preparation of breakfast encourages children to eat better. Making pancakes or French toast, preparing scrambled eggs, and squeezing fresh orange juice are all within the capabilities of young children with a little help from Mom or Dad.

Meal planner

	BREAKFAST	LUNCH	SUPPER
DAY 1	Boiled or fried egg with fingers of toast Yogurt Fruit	Tuna Tortilla Roll-ups (page 170) Fruit	My Favorite Beefburgers (page 166) with vegetables Heavenly Chocolate Mini Cakes (page 175)
DAY 2	Cereal Cheese Stewed prunes	Diced Chicken in Lettuce with Plum Sauce (page 158) Strawberry Sorbet Ice Pops (page 178)	Spinach, Cheese, and Tomato Lasagne (page 171) Fruit and ice cream
DAY 3	Apple, Oat, and Raisin Muffins (page 182) Yogurt Fruit	Mini Vegetable Burgers (page 172) Fruit	New England Seafood Potpies (page 169) Mixed Berry and Peach Crumble (page 174)
DAY 4	Scrambled egg with toast Fruit	Chicken Fingers Marinated in Buttermilk (page 156) with oven fries and vegetables Fruit	Thai-Style Chicken and Noodles (page 159) Fruit
DAY 5	Grilled cheese on toast Fruit	Tofu and Vegetable Burgers (page 170) Dark and White Chocolate Refrigerator Cake (page 178)	Stir-fried Shredded Beef (page 167) Cranberry, Lemonade, and Orange Juice Ice Pops (page 179)
DAY 6	Pancake/waffle with maple syrup Yogurt Fruit	Cheesy Baked Potato with Butternut Squash (page 132) Fruit and ice cream	Mini Veal Schnitzel with Rösti (page 163) with vegetables Fruit
DAY 7	Oatmeal with honey or jam Cheese Fruit	Marinated Lamb Chops (page 163) with vegetables Summer Fruit Milkshake (page 183)	Delicious Chicken Fajitas (page 164) Cranberry-Raspberry Gelatin with Summer Fruits (page 180)

Include three servings of dairy products daily, such as cheese, yogurt, and a milk-based drink.

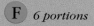
SUPERFOODS

Ginger *aids digestion and is also a good remedy for nausea, particularly travel sickness. Grated fresh gingerroot in a hot lemon and honey drink can help alleviate the symptoms of a cold. Mix together the juice of half a lemon, some grated fresh gingerroot, and a teaspoon or two of honey in a mug and pour in boiling water.*

Healthy eating:

If you don't want to make your own chicken stock, you can buy some good fresh chicken stock in cartons in large supermarkets.

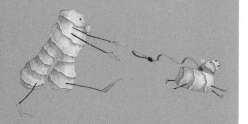

Chicken noodle soup

1 boneless, skinless chicken breast

MARINADE
2 tablespoons soy sauce
1 teaspoon Asian sesame oil
½ teaspoon grated fresh gingerroot
1 tablespoon honey
1 clove garlic, crushed

4 cups chicken stock
4 ounces egg noodles
1 cup frozen or canned corn
3 scallions, thinly sliced

Slice the chicken breast in half to make two thin fillets. Mix all the ingredients for the marinade and marinate the chicken for 30 minutes; remove the chicken and reserve the marinade.

Bring the stock to a boil, then reduce the heat to low (barely simmering) and cook the chicken for about 20 minutes or until cooked through. Remove the chicken with a slotted spoon and allow to cool down slightly. Then shred the chicken very fine.

Cook the noodles according to the package instructions. Stir the corn, scallions, and reserved marinade into the stock. Bring to a boil, then add the shredded chicken and noodles and heat through.

Nasi goreng

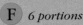
Nasi goreng is a traditional Indonesian rice dish. It is usually made with roasted peanuts, and if you like, you can scatter 2 tablespoons of roasted peanuts on top before serving.

1 cup long-grain rice
Vegetable oil for frying
4 shallots, cut into very fine rings, or 2 small onions, sliced

OMELET
1 egg
Salt

STIR-FRY
1 boneless, skinless chicken breast, cut into small strips
1 clove garlic, crushed
Pinch of mild chili powder
4 ounces cooked shrimp, peeled
4 scallions, sliced
2 tablespoons soy sauce
1 tablespoon chopped fresh parsley

Cook the rice according to the package instructions and allow to cool. Heat 1 inch of oil in a small frying pan. To test if it is hot enough, drop a piece of shallot into the oil. If it sizzles and bubbles, the oil is ready. Sauté the shallots in two batches until golden brown (1 to 2 minutes) and drain on paper towels.

To make the omelet, beat the egg with a pinch of salt and ½ teaspoon water. Heat 1 teaspoon of the oil in a frying pan. Pour in the egg and swirl to thinly cover the base of the pan. Cook for about 1 minute or until set, then turn over and cook for 30 seconds on the other side. Remove from the pan and cut into strips.

Heat 2 tablespoons of the vegetable oil in a wok or frying pan and stir-fry the chicken and garlic for 3 to 4 minutes. Stir in the chili powder, shrimp, and scallions and stir-fry for about 2 minutes. Add the rice and stir in the soy sauce and parsley and stir-fry for 4 to 5 minutes. Finally, stir in the strips of egg and golden shallots.

Shrimp *is an excellent source of vitamin B_{12}, which is necessary for the formation of blood cells and nerves, and also provides selenium, which is important for growth and helps protect against heart disease and cancer.*

SUPERFOODS

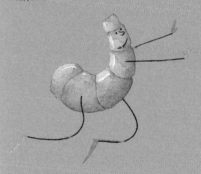

Chicken *is a good, high-quality source of protein. The body is approximately 25 percent protein; it is needed for all our cells and muscles and helps children to grow big and strong. Chicken also contains vitamins B_3 and B_6, which the body needs for converting the food we eat into energy.*

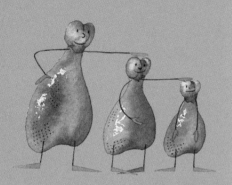

Chicken fingers marinated in buttermilk

Marinating chicken in buttermilk gives it a lovely flavor and makes it very tender.

2 boneless, skinless chicken breasts
Salt and freshly ground black pepper
1 cup buttermilk
1 tablespoon lemon juice
1 teaspoon Worcestershire sauce
1 teaspoon soy sauce
¼ teaspoon paprika
1 clove garlic, sliced
¾ cup dried bread crumbs or fresh white bread crumbs
3 tablespoons sesame seeds
Vegetable oil for frying

Cut each chicken breast into ½-inch strips and season with salt and pepper. Combine the buttermilk, lemon juice, Worcestershire sauce, soy sauce, paprika, and garlic in a bowl. Add the chicken strips and toss to coat. Cover and refrigerate for at least 1 hour or ovenight.

    Drain the chicken well. In a large bowl, toss the breadcrumbs with the sesame seeds and some salt and pepper. Heat the oil in a large frying pan. Roll the chicken strips in the crumbs to coat and sauté until golden and cooked through, turning occasionally.

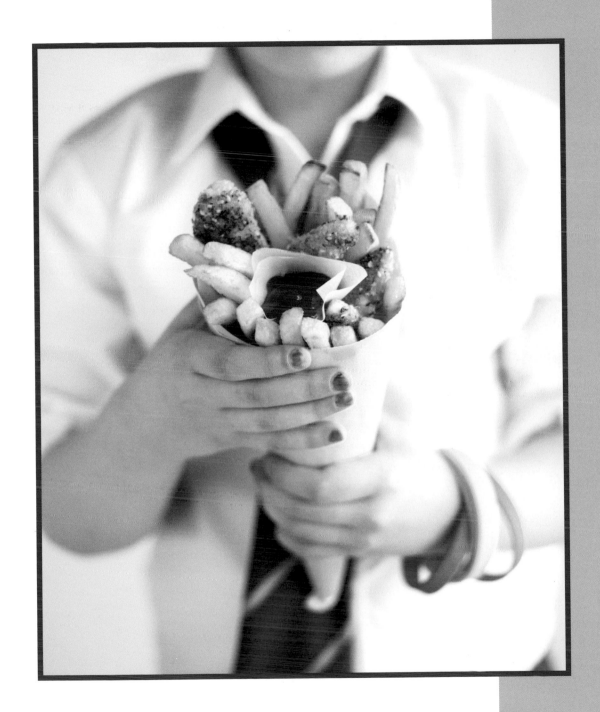

SUPERFOODS

Lettuce *is rich in vitamins A and C, potassium, calcium, and folic acid. The darker the lettuce leaves, the more nutrients they contain. Lettuce also contains phytochemicals that act as a mild sedative and may help induce sleep. Always remove and discard the outer leaves of lettuce.*

Diced chicken in lettuce with plum sauce

I think it's really important to make food fun for children and I find that they really enjoy assembling food. The crunchy lettuce, soft diced chicken, and vegetables with sweet plum sauce make this a winning combination. Fingers only, please! If you can't find plum jam, you can simply use a jar of prepared plum sauce, which is readily available in the Asian section of most supermarkets.

1 tablespoon all-purpose flour
¼ teaspoon ground ginger
¼ teaspoon mild curry powder
Salt and freshly ground black pepper
1 large boneless, skinless chicken breast, diced
1 tablespoon vegetable oil
1 clove garlic, crushed
½ medium onion, chopped
1 medium carrot, peeled and finely diced
1 small zucchini, finely diced
¼ cup chicken stock

PLUM SAUCE
¼ cup plum jam
1 tablespoon soy sauce
¼ teaspoon mild chili powder
2 teaspoons rice wine vinegar or white wine vinegar

Iceberg or Boston lettuce

Mix together the flour, ginger, curry powder, and salt and pepper and then stir in the diced chicken to coat with the spices. Heat the oil in a wok or frying pan and sauté the garlic and onion for 2 minutes. Add the carrot and cook for another minute, then stir in the chicken and sauté for 4 minutes, stirring frequently. Add the zucchini and cook for 1 minute. Then stir in the chicken stock and cook until thickened (about 2 minutes).

To make the plum sauce, place all of the ingredients in a small pan over low heat. Stir until the jam has melted. Strain through a sieve and set aside to cool slightly.

Spoon the chicken mixture into lettuce leaves and top with a little plum sauce. Wrap up to form small packages.

Thai-style chicken and noodles

4 portions

This is a delicious recipe flavored with peanut butter and coconut milk. It makes a great meal for the whole family and is very quick to prepare.

1 tablespoon sunflower oil

1 medium onion, finely chopped

2 large boneless, skinless chicken breasts, cut into strips

1 cup chopped broccoli florets

1/2 teaspoon chopped green chile

1 cup unsweetened coconut milk

1/4 cup peanut butter

Juice of 1/2 lime

1 tablespoon soy sauce

1/2 cup chicken stock

1 cup bean sprouts

6 ounces Chinese cellophane noodles (bean threads)

Heat the oil in a pan or wok and sauté the onion for 4 minutes. Add the chicken, broccoli, and chile and stir-fry for about 3 minutes. Stir in the coconut milk, peanut butter, lime juice, soy sauce, chicken stock, and bean sprouts. Bring to a simmer, stirring until the peanut butter has melted, and cook for 3 to 4 minutes. Meanwhile, soak the noodles in boiling water according to the package instructions. Drain the noodles and toss with the sauce.

Peanut butter *is a nutrient-dense and energy-giving food, providing an excellent source of protein, folic acid, calcium, and zinc. Zinc plays an important role in building up a strong immune system.*

SUPERFOODS

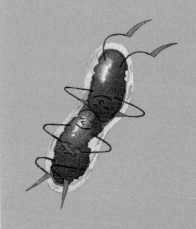

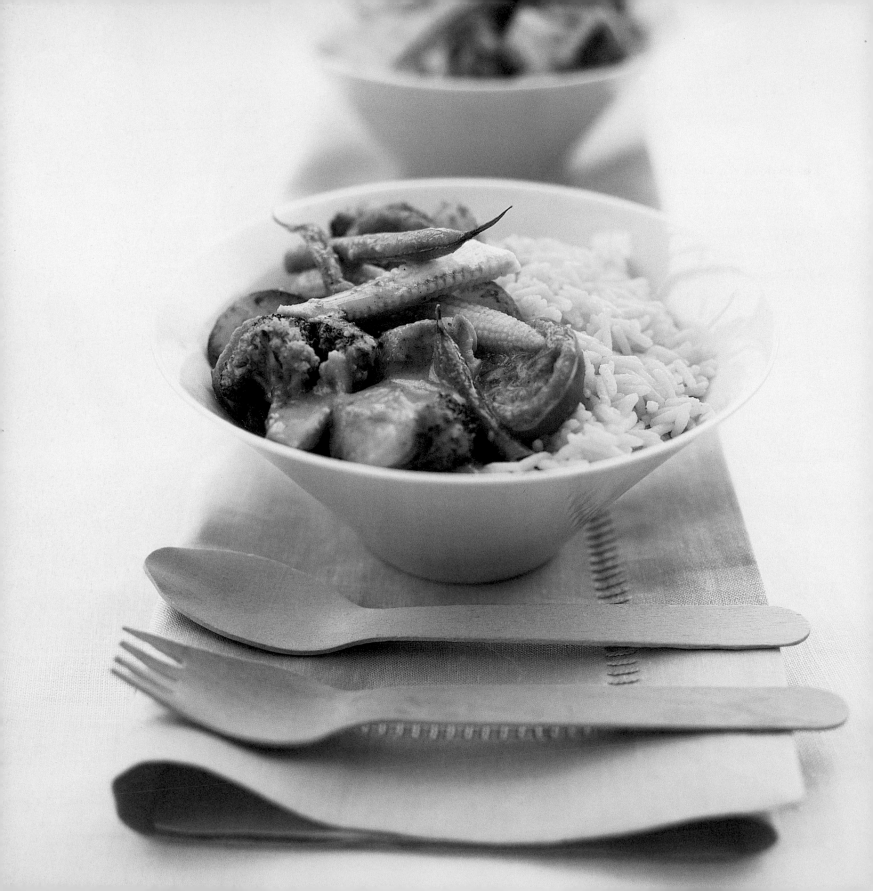

Thai-style chicken curry

A really tasty quick and easy curry.

1 tablespoon vegetable oil

2 large boneless, skinless chicken breasts, cut into strips

1 large new potato, scrubbed and thinly sliced

One 15-ounce can unsweetened coconut milk

2 teaspoons green Thai curry paste

2 cups chicken stock

¼ cup green beans, trimmed and cut in half

6 whole baby corn

1 cup chopped broccoli florets

12 cherry tomatoes, halved

1 teaspoon superfine sugar

1 teaspoon lime or lemon juice

Heat the oil in a wok or large frying pan and fry the chicken and potato until the chicken turns opaque (3 to 4 minutes). Stir in the coconut milk, curry paste, and chicken stock. Bring to a simmer and cook for 5 to 6 minutes, then add the beans, whole baby corn, and broccoli. Simmer until the vegetables are tender (another 8 to 10 minutes). Stir in the cherry tomatoes, sugar, and lime or lemon juice.

Healthy eating:

Many children's diets can be rather unadventurous, consisting of the usual burgers, pizzas, and chicken nuggets. Introduce children to a wide variety of flavors so they don't grow up to be fussy eaters. Mild curry is often very popular, particularly when it is combined with coconut milk, as here.

Pilau rice

This rice has a wonderful flavor, and the turmeric turns the rice a rich yellow color, which is very attractive.

1 cup basmati rice

1 tablespoon butter

½ teaspoon ground turmeric

2 cardamom pods

2 cloves

½ cinnamon stick

1½ cups boiling water

Salt

Rinse the rice until the water runs clear through a sieve.

In a medium saucepan, melt the butter and stir in the rice and spices until evenly coated in butter. Stir in the boiling water and a pinch of salt. Cover and leave to cook on the lowest heat for 10 minutes. Remove from the heat and leave in the pan, without uncovering or stirring, for 10 minutes. Remove the cardamom, cloves, and cinnamon stick, and fluff up with a fork.

Spices *have specific health benefits. It is believed that cardamom, for example, can relieve indigestion and aid coughs and colds. Cinnamon can help indigestion and diarrhea and relieve nasal congestion, and turmeric can help calm inflammation and relieve indigestion.*

SUPERFOODS

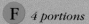 **F** *4 portions*

SUPERFOODS

Ketchup *requires 25 tomatoes to fill one bottle. Lycopene, the natural red pigment found in tomatoes, has been linked with a lower risk of prostate cancer and heart disease. Although nutritionists emphasize the benefits of fresh fruits and vegetables, lycopene is easier for our bodies to absorb when the tomatoes have been cooked or processed with a little oil into foods such as ketchup or pasta sauce.*

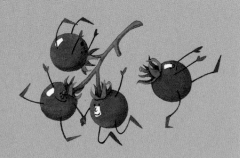

Chicken cannelloni

Decorating these tasty cannelloni to look like people sleeping in a bed will add oodles of child appeal (see Spinach and Ricotta Cannelloni on page 127). Older children will love to help.

CHICKEN AND TOMATO FILLING

1 medium onion, chopped

1 small clove garlic, crushed

1 tablespoon olive oil

1/2 cup chopped button mushrooms

1/2 teaspoon dried mixed herbs,
   such as Italian Seasoning

8 ounces ground chicken

1 cup canned chopped tomatoes

1 1/2 teaspoons ketchup

CHEESE SAUCE

2 tablespoons butter

2 tablespoons all-purpose flour

1/2 teaspoon paprika

1 2/3 cups whole milk

1 cup grated Cheddar cheese

8 no-boil cannelloni or lasagne sheets

Sauté the onion and garlic for 2 minutes in the oil. Then add the mushrooms, herbs, and chicken and sauté for 3 minutes. Stir in the chopped tomatoes and ketchup and simmer for 20 minutes.

To make the cheese sauce, melt the butter, stir in the flour and paprika, and cook for 1 minute. Gradually whisk in the milk. Bring to a boil and then simmer, stirring, until thickened. Stir in half the grated cheese.

Preheat the oven to 350°F. Stuff the cannelloni with the chicken and tomato filling and arrange them in a shallow ovenproof dish. Pour in the cheese sauce, sprinkle with the remaining cheese, and bake in the oven for 25 minutes.

Mini veal schnitzel with rösti

The veal is also good marinated in lemon juice, olive oil, or garlic, and sautéed.

4 veal scallops, about 10 ounces total

Salt and freshly ground black pepper

1 tablespoon lemon juice

All-purpose flour for coating

1 egg, lightly beaten

Seasoned bread crumbs

Vegetable oil for frying

ROSTI

1 onion

1 pound potatoes, peeled

1 clove garlic, crushed

Salt and freshly ground black pepper

4 tablespoons butter, melted

Place the veal scallops between sheets of plastic wrap and flatten with a mallet until they are quite thin. Season with salt, pepper, and the lemon juice and then coat in flour. Dip in the egg and then into the seasoned bread crumbs. Sauté the scallops in a skillet in vegetable oil for 2 to 3 minutes on each side.

For the rösti, grate the onion and potatoes, then mix with the crushed garlic and season with salt and pepper. Take a small handful, squeeze out the excess liquid, and sauté in a skillet in the melted butter for 3 to 4 minutes on each side.

4 portions

Veal *is a good source of protein, vitamin B_{12}, and zinc and contains just under half the fat of lean red meat. This recipe could also be made successfully with chicken breasts.*

Marinated lamb chops

Children love lamb chops. Some prefer you to trim the fat and cut the meat into bite-size bits.

MARINADE

2 teaspoons lemon juice

1 teaspoon soy sauce

1 teaspoon Asian sesame oil

½ teaspoon herbes de Provence or
   other dried mixed herbs,
   such as Italian Seasoning

1 teaspoon light brown sugar

Pinch of salt

Freshly ground black pepper

4 lamb chops

Combine the marinade ingredients and marinate the lamb for at least 1 hour in the refrigerator. Remove the lamb from the marinade and broil for about 8 minutes, turning the lamb halfway through and basting occasionally. Boil any remaining marinade and pour over the lamb chops.

4 portions

Red meat and lamb *provide the best source of iron, followed by pork and chicken. Lamb contains all the essential amino acids needed for growth and repair of tissue damage. Children grow so quickly they need regular high-protein foods. For young children, cut the lamb into small cubes and remove all the fat.*

SUPERFOODS

SUPERFOODS

Chicken *is a good source of lean protein and has the advantage of being very versatile and quick to cook. The darker the meat of the chicken, the more fat it contains, and the skin is very high in fat, too.*

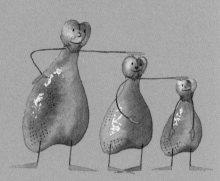

Delicious chicken fajitas

These are a great favorite of mine and I have made them much less hot and spicy so that children will enjoy eating them. My children love to assemble these and roll them up themselves. Everything can be prepared in advance.

2 small boneless, skinless chicken breasts, cut into strips
⅛ teaspoon paprika
⅛ teaspoon mild chili powder
⅛ teaspoon ground cumin (optional)
¼ teaspoon dried oregano
1 tablespoon plus 1 teaspoon olive oil
1 clove garlic, crushed
1 medium onion, thinly sliced
½ small red bell pepper, seeded and thinly sliced
Salt and freshly ground black pepper

TOMATO SALSA
1½ teaspoons olive oil
¼ green chile, finely sliced
½ medium onion, chopped
½ small green bell pepper, seeded and diced
1 small clove garlic, finely chopped
½ teaspoon red wine vinegar
1 cup canned chopped tomatoes
Salt and freshly ground black pepper
1½ teaspoons chopped fresh parsley

8 small flour tortillas
1 cup shredded iceberg lettuce
1 cup grated Cheddar cheese
3 tablespoons sour cream

Toss the chicken in the paprika, chili powder, cumin (if using), and oregano. Heat the 1 teaspoon oil in a pan and sauté the chicken, stirring occasionally, for 3 to 4 minutes. Remove the chicken with a slotted spoon. Add the 1 tablespoon oil and sauté the garlic, onion, and red pepper for 5 minutes. Return the chicken to the pan, season to taste, and heat through.

To make the tomato salsa, heat the oil and fry the chile, onion, green pepper, and garlic for about 5 minutes. Add the vinegar and cook for about 20 seconds. Add the chopped tomatoes, salt and pepper, and parsley and simmer, uncovered, for about 15 minutes.

To assemble, heat the tortillas in a microwave according to the package instructions. Then place some of the chicken mixture along the center of each tortilla, top with some tomato salsa, shredded lettuce, grated cheese, and a little sour cream, and roll up.

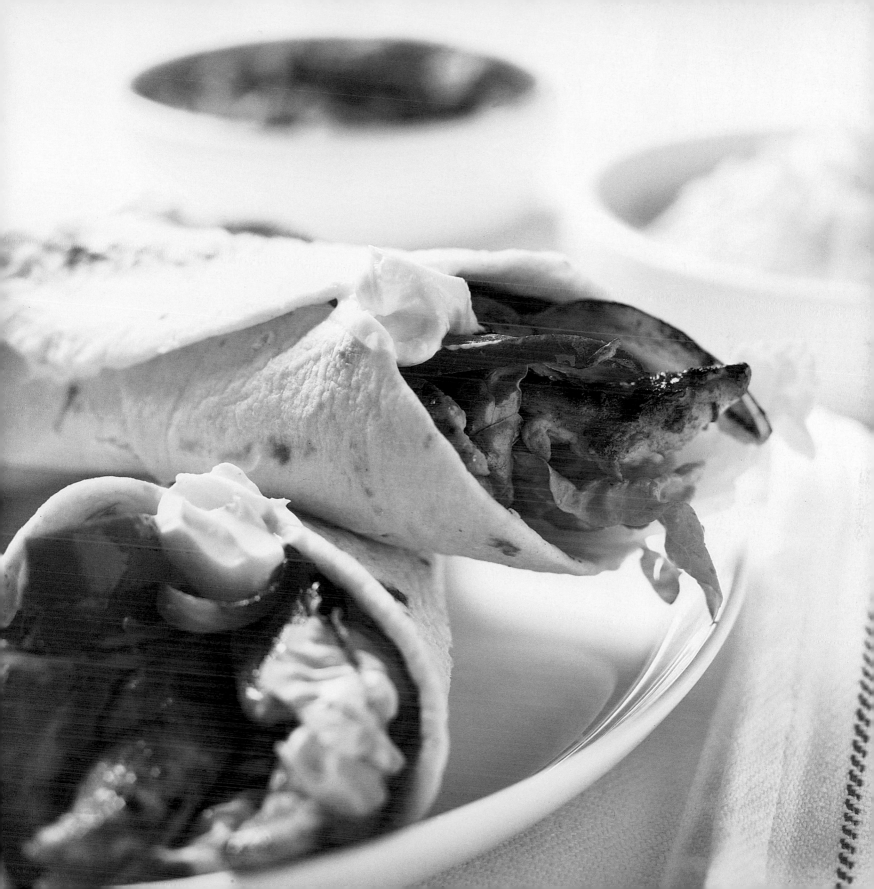

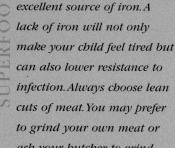

SUPERFOODS

Ground beef *is an excellent source of iron. A lack of iron will not only make your child feel tired but can also lower resistance to infection. Always choose lean cuts of meat. You may prefer to grind your own meat or ask your butcher to grind some good cuts for you.*

Warning: *Undercooked burgers may contain harmful bacteria such as E. coli.*

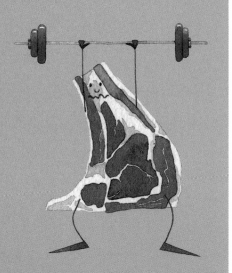

F *10 burgers*

My favorite beefburgers

My secret ingredient in these burgers is grated apple, which gives them a lovely flavor and keeps them moist. Make fresh bread crumbs by blitzing slices of white bread in a food processor. Serve these with or without the barbecue sauce.

1 medium onion, finely chopped
½ red bell pepper, seeded and chopped
Vegetable oil for frying
1 pound ground beef, lamb, or chicken
2 tablespoons finely chopped fresh parsley
1 chicken bouillon cube, finely crumbled
1 cup fresh bread crumbs
1 Granny Smith apple, peeled and grated
Salt and freshly ground black pepper
1 egg, beaten

All-purpose flour

BARBECUE SAUCE
2 tablespoons vegetable oil
1 small red onion, diced
1 clove garlic, crushed
1 cup canned crushed tomatoes
1 tablespoon tomato paste
2 tablespoons white wine vinegar
2 tablespoons dark brown sugar
1½ teaspoons Worcestershire sauce
Few drops of Tabasco

Rolls, lettuce, sliced tomato

Sauté the onion and red pepper in a small amount of vegetable oil until soft (about 5 minutes). Combine with all the other burger ingredients and, using your hands, form into about 10 burgers and lightly coat with flour. Fry until browned and cooked through (about 5 minutes per side). Alternatively, cook the burgers under a preheated broiler or on a barbecue.

For the sauce, heat the oil in a small pan and sauté the onion for 8 minutes. Add the garlic and sauté for 1 minute. Add the remaining ingredients for the sauce, cover, and simmer for about 8 minutes. Puree with a hand blender to make a smooth sauce. Serve the burgers on rolls with lettuce, tomato slices, and the barbecue sauce.

Stir-fried shredded beef

1 tablespoon Asian sesame oil

1 clove garlic, crushed

1 medium carrot, peeled and cut
into matchsticks

1 small zucchini, cut into matchsticks

1/2 yellow bell pepper, seeded and
cut into matchsticks

10 ounces tender beef fillet,
cut into very fine strips

1 tablespoon cornstarch

1/2 cup beef stock

2 tablespoons dark brown sugar

2 tablespoons soy sauce

Few drops of Tabasco

1 tablespoon sesame seeds

Heat the sesame oil in a wok. Stir-fry the garlic, carrot, zucchini, and pepper for 3 to 4 minutes. Add the beef and stir-fry for 4 to 5 minutes. Mix the cornstarch with 1 tablespoon of water and stir into the beef stock. Stir this into the pan with the sugar, soy sauce, Tabasco, and sesame seeds. Bring to a simmer, cook until slightly thickened, and serve with rice.

SUPERFOODS

 Red meat *is packed full of high-quality protein as well as being the best source of easily absorbed iron. It is also a good source of zinc and vitamin B_{12}.*

Mild beef curry

Young children often have more sophisticated tastes than we give them credit for and it's important to introduce lots of variety at a young age when children are more likely to accept new tastes. Children will love this curry. Serve with Pilau Rice (page 161).

1 tablespoon vegetable oil

2 medium onions, chopped

1 clove garlic, crushed

1/2 teaspoon grated fresh gingerroot

1 pound stewing beef (blade or round),
cut into 1-inch cubes

2 tablespoons mild curry powder

1 green bell pepper, seeded and
cut into 1-inch pieces

1 cup beef stock

2 tablespoons tomato paste

1 cup heavy cream

1 tablespoon ground almonds

Salt and freshly ground black pepper

3 tomatoes, peeled, seeded, and chopped

Heat the oil in a large saucepan. Fry the onions, garlic, and gingerroot until softened (5 to 6 minutes). Stir in the beef and curry powder and cook until the meat is browned (2 to 3 minutes). Stir in the pepper and cook for 1 minute. Stir in the stock, tomato paste, cream, and almonds; season with salt and pepper. Bring to a boil and simmer for 45 minutes, then stir in the tomatoes and cook until thickened (10 to 15 minutes). Taste and adjust seasoning.

SUPERFOODS

Red meat *provides the best source of iron, which is important for healthy red blood cells. Children need increasing amounts of iron, as they grow so rapidly. The brain is the largest store of iron and it is essential that adequate iron is present in the diet to support good brain development.*

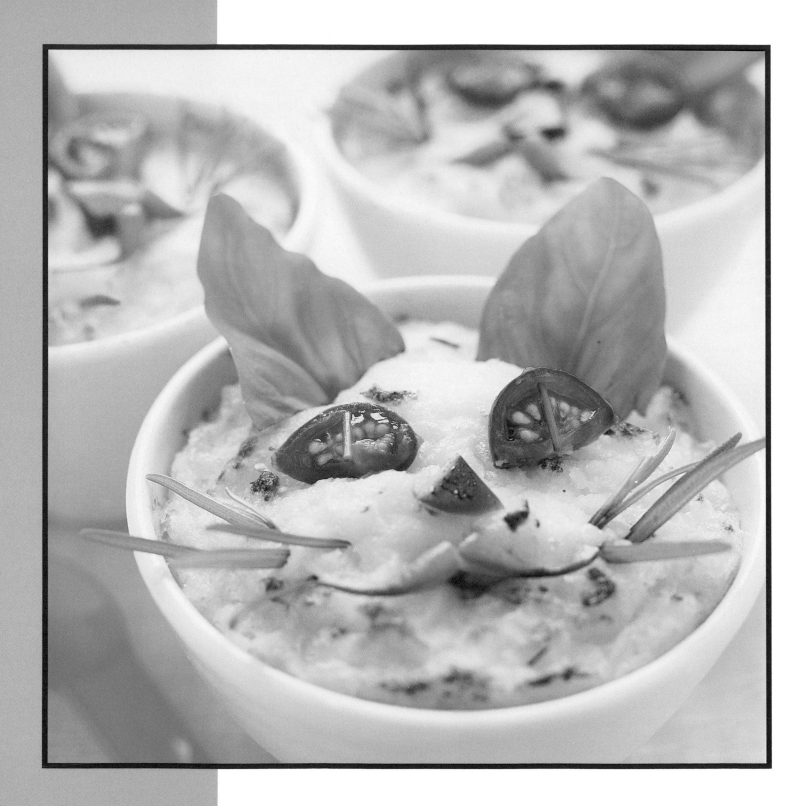

New England seafood potpies

This is a really tasty recipe for an old-fashioned favorite. It also looks good prepared in layers in a glass ovenproof dish. First make a layer of the scallops, shrimp, and sauce, then add a layer of fish with the sauce, next a layer of peas, and finally top with the mashed potato.

Fish *is such a wonderful nutrient-dense food that it is important to find tasty recipes for fish that children will enjoy. This is very popular with my three children and Daddy's quite partial to it, too!*

SUPERFOODS

2 pounds potatoes, peeled and cut into chunks
10 ounces haddock, cod, scrod, salmon, or whitefish fillets, skinned and cut into chunks
2¼ cups whole milk
6 peppercorns
1 bay leaf
1 parsley sprig
6 tablespoons butter
⅓ pound scallops

⅓ pound shrimp, peeled and deveined (alternatively use ⅔ pound scallops or shrimp)
1 medium onion, finely chopped
3 tablespoons all-purpose flour
⅓ cup grated Cheddar cheese
White pepper
1⅓ cups frozen peas
1 egg, lightly beaten

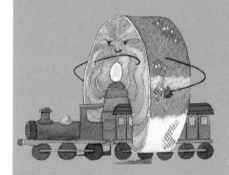

Preheat the oven to 350°F. For the mashed potatoes, boil some lightly salted water, add the potatoes, and boil until tender.

Meanwhile, put the fish chunks in a shallow pan with 2 cups of the milk, the peppercorns, and the herbs. Bring to a boil, then reduce the heat, cover, and simmer for 5 minutes or until the fish flakes easily. Remove the fish; strain the milk (discard the peppercorns and herbs), and reserve. Flake the fish with a fork, checking carefully for bones, and set aside.

Melt 2 tablespoons of the butter in a pan and sauté the scallops and shrimp for 2 minutes. Remove with a slotted spoon, then cut in half. Melt another 2 tablespoons of the butter in a separate pan, add the onion, and sauté until softened. Stir in the flour to make a paste and cook for 1 minute. Gradually add the reserved milk, stirring until the sauce thickens. Remove from the heat and stir in the cheese until melted. Season to taste with salt and white pepper, then stir in the frozen peas. Spoon the fish into four ramekins.

Drain and mash the potatoes. Add the remaining ¼ cup milk and the remaining 2 tablespoons butter, and season to taste. Spread the potatoes over the fish in the ramekins, making lines on the surface using a fork. Brush with the beaten egg.

Bake for 15 to 20 minutes and finish off under a broiler until browned on top.

If you like, you can decorate the potpies with faces made from vegetables

Canned tuna *is a good source of vitamins, especially vitamins D and B$_{12}$. It is also a good source of the anti-oxidant selenium, which helps to protect us against heart disease and cancer. Eating an oily fish like tuna once a week has been shown to reduce heart disease.*

Tuna tortilla roll-ups

One 6-ounce can tuna in oil
1½ tablespoons mayonnaise
¾ teaspoon lemon juice
¼ teaspoon paprika
⅔ cup frozen or canned corn
  (cook if frozen)

¼ cup thinly sliced cucumber, red bell
  pepper, or celery
2 small tortillas
Shredded iceberg lettuce
2 chives (optional)

Drain the tuna and mix together with the mayonnaise, lemon juice, and paprika. Stir in the corn and cucumber, red pepper, or celery. Place the tuna mixture along the center of each tortilla. Cover with some shredded lettuce and roll up. You can secure each tortilla by tying a chive around it.

Nuts *are great for vegetarians, as they supply many of the nutrients usually found in animal sources. Combining cashew nuts with tofu, as in this recipe, makes for a good source of protein. Cashew nuts, like olive oil, are rich in heart-protecting monounsaturated fats.*

Tofu and vegetable burgers

BURGERS
1 cup chopped broccoli florets
1 tablespoon butter
2½ cups roughly chopped
  button mushrooms
1 clove garlic, crushed
10 ounces firm tofu
¼ cup unsalted cashew nuts
3 scallions, finely sliced

1 medium carrot, peeled and
  finely grated
1 cup fresh bread crumbs
1 tablespoon oyster sauce
1 tablespoon honey

Salt and freshly ground black pepper
All-purpose flour for coating
Vegetable oil for frying

Blanch the broccoli in lightly salted boiling water until tender (about 2 minutes). Melt the butter in a frying pan and sauté the mushrooms and garlic until softened (3 to 4 minutes). Transfer to a food processor with the broccoli and all the other burger ingredients. Process until mixed together and season with salt and pepper.

Form into eight burgers, coat in flour, and sauté in vegetable oil in a skillet over medium heat until golden (2 to 3 minutes on each side).

Spinach, cheese, and tomato lasagne

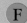 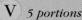 5 portions

The good thing about making a lasagne is that you can hide lots of vegetables inside it.

TOMATO SAUCE

2 tablespoons olive oil

1 large onion, chopped

2 pounds plum tomatoes, peeled, seeded, and chopped, or one 28-ounce can chopped tomatoes

1 clove garlic, crushed

¼ cup vegetable stock

2 tablespoons tomato paste

1 teaspoon superfine sugar

1 bay leaf

1 teaspoon balsamic vinegar

6 basil leaves, roughly torn

Salt and freshly ground black pepper

CHEESE SAUCE

3 tablespoons butter

⅓ cup all-purpose flour

1⅔ cups whole milk

Generous pinch of ground nutmeg

½ cup grated Gruyère cheese

½ cup grated Cheddar cheese

Salt and freshly ground black pepper

1 pound fresh baby spinach, carefully washed, or one 10-ounce package frozen leaf spinach

9 sheets fresh or no-boil lasagne

3 tablespoons grated Parmesan cheese

To make the tomato sauce, heat the oil in a large saucepan and sauté the onion for 2 to 3 minutes. Stir in the tomatoes and garlic, bring to a simmer, and stir in the vegetable stock, tomato paste, sugar, bay leaf, and balsamic vinegar. Cover and simmer for 20 minutes. Remove the lid and simmer to thicken the sauce for an additional 10 minutes. Remove the bay leaf, stir in the basil, and season to taste.

To make the cheese sauce, melt the butter in a saucepan. Stir in the flour and cook for 1 minute over low heat. Gradually whisk in the milk and nutmeg, bring to a boil, and then cook for 1 minute or until thickened and smooth. Remove from the heat and stir in the grated cheeses until melted. Season with salt and pepper.

Cook the spinach in a large pan with just a little water clinging to the leaves until wilted (about 3 minutes). Gently press out any excess liquid and roughly chop the spinach.

Preheat the oven to 350°F. Spread a little of the cheese sauce in an 11 x 7-inch or 13 x 9-inch lasagne dish and cover with three sheets of lasagne (break up the third sheet to fit if necessary). Arrange half the spinach over the lasagne and top with one-third of the cheese sauce and half the tomato sauce. Arrange another layer of lasagne on top and repeat with the spinach, cheese sauce, and tomato sauce. Arrange a third layer of lasagne and spread the remainder of the cheese sauce over the pasta to cover it completely. Sprinkle the top with the grated Parmesan and bake for 30 minutes. Brown under the broiler for a few minutes.

SUPERFOODS

Basil *can aid digestion, easing the symptoms of gas, stomach cramps, colic, and indigestion.*

Healthy eating:
Fresh basil and tomato are perfect partners in this delicious lasagne, which makes a popular family meal. Always tear basil leaves rather than cut them to preserve their flavor.

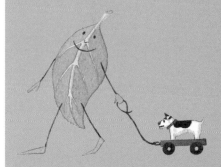

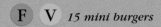

Onions and leeks

have a protective action on the circulatory system that helps to prevent blood clots. With children eating more and more junk food, fatty deposits in the arteries can now be found in even the youngest children, and in later life these deposits may lead to heart disease, as will arterial blood clots. When fat deposits and blood clots break loose and clog the arteries, the result is a heart attack or stroke.

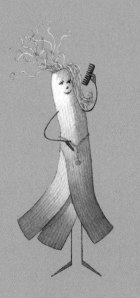

Mini vegetable burgers

These tasty mini burgers in a crispy coating are bursting with fresh vegetables and flavored with Gruyère cheese.

2 medium potatoes (do not peel)
2 tablespoons butter
1 small onion, chopped
½ cup chopped broccoli florets
½ cup grated carrot
½ cup washed and finely chopped white part of a leek
1 cup chopped button mushrooms
1 cup frozen or canned corn
1 teaspoon soy sauce
¾ cup grated Gruyère cheese
1 tablespoon chopped fresh parsley
Cayenne pepper
Salt and freshly ground black pepper
Seasoned all-purpose flour (flour mixed with a little salt and pepper)
2 eggs, lightly beaten
1 cup bread crumbs
Vegetable oil for frying

15 mini buns
Lettuce
Ketchup

Cook the potatoes in a pan of boiling water for 25 to 30 minutes, then peel and grate. Meanwhile, melt the butter and sauté the onion for about 3 minutes. Add the broccoli, carrot, leek, and mushrooms, and sauté for 5 minutes. Add the grated potato, corn, soy sauce, cheese, parsley, a pinch of cayenne pepper, and salt and pepper to taste. Form the mixture into 15 mini burgers, coat with flour, dip in the beaten egg, and then dip in the bread crumbs. Dip in the egg once again and then coat with another layer of bread crumbs to make a crispy coating for the burgers. Sauté in a small amount of oil in a skillet until crisp and golden on both sides. Serve on their own or in mini buns with a little lettuce and ketchup.

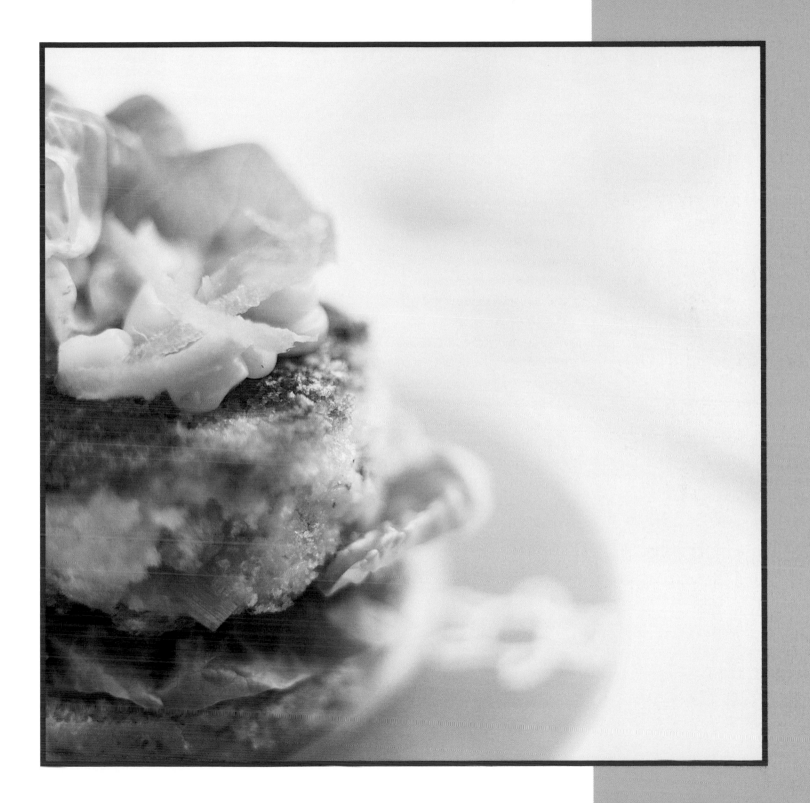

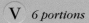

Berries *are rich in vitamin C, which is important for growth, wound healing, and healthy skin.*

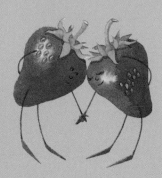

Mixed berry and peach crumble

Here is a truly delicious crumble made from mixed frozen berries and canned peaches. I put a layer of ground almonds into the baking dish before I spoon in the summer berries to soak up some of the juices that are released from the fruit during cooking so that they do not bubble over the topping and make it soggy. Serve hot on its own or with ice cream or whipped cream.

TOPPING

1 cup all-purpose flour
1 cup rolled oats
¾ cup light brown sugar
Pinch of salt
1 stick butter

¼ cup ground almonds
One 15-ounce can peaches
2 cups fresh or one 12-ounce package frozen mixed berries, such as raspberries, blackberries, strawberries, and blueberries
1 cup superfine sugar

Preheat the oven to 400°F. To make the topping, mix together the flour, oats, brown sugar, and salt. Cut the butter into pieces and rub in with your fingers until the mixture resembles coarse bread crumbs. Spread the ground almonds over the base of an 8-inch round ovenproof dish. Mix the peaches and berries together with the superfine sugar and spoon into the dish. Sprinkle the topping over the fruit and bake until golden (about 30 minutes).

Heavenly mini chocolate cakes

V *4 portions*

These are individual warm chocolate cakes with melted chocolate centers. You can prepare the batter several hours ahead, refrigerate, and then bring back to room temperature before baking. Serve hot with a scoop of vanilla ice cream and some fresh raspberries. You can also freeze the uncooked batter.

1 stick unsalted butter, cut into pieces, plus extra for greasing
¾ cup all-purpose flour, plus extra for dusting
¼ pound good-quality semisweet chocolate, broken into pieces
2 whole eggs
2 egg yolks
¾ cup superfine sugar
Confectioners' sugar for dusting
Vanilla ice cream
Fresh raspberries

Preheat the oven to 400°F. Place a baking sheet in the oven to heat. Grease four ramekins or individual metal baking dishes with butter and dust lightly with flour. Put the chocolate and butter into a heatproof bowl and melt over a pan of simmering water, making sure that the bowl doesn't touch the hot water. Stir occasionally until melted.

Beat the whole eggs, yolks, and sugar for about 5 minutes with an electric mixer until thickened and pale. Gradually fold the melted chocolate mixture into the eggs. Fold in the ¾ cup flour. Pour the mixture into the ramekins and place on the hot baking sheet. Bake for about 10 minutes or until firm around the edges. Allow to cool for a few minutes, run a knife around the sides of the ramekins, and turn out onto serving plates. Dust with confectioners' sugar. Serve with a scoop of vanilla ice cream and some fresh raspberries.

Chocolate

manufacturers in the United States use about 3.5 million pounds of whole milk every day to make chocolate. The melting point of cocoa butter is just below the temperature of the human body, which is why chocolate literally melts in the mouth. More than $1 billion in boxed chocolate is sold between Thanksgiving and New Year's.

It's no surprise that love and chocolate go hand in hand: Phenylethylamine, a naturally occurring organic compound that promotes the feeling of euphoria associated with being in love, is found in chocolate.

Chocolate is surprisingly nutritious, containing iron, calcium, and potassium plus vitamins A, B_1, C, D, and E. Ten percent of the USDA recommended daily allowance of iron is found in 1 ounce of baking chocolate.

SUPERFOODS

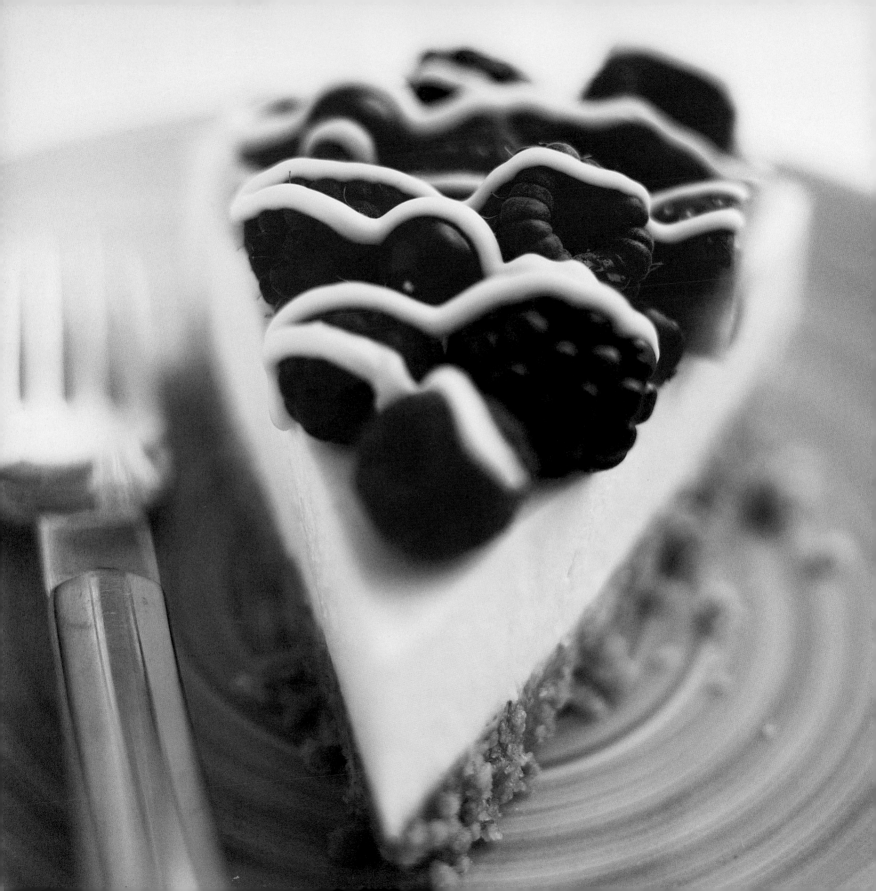

Mixed berry and white chocolate cheesecake

F V *8 portions*

CRUMB CRUST

8 ounces graham crackers (2½ cups crumbs)

1 stick butter, melted

Vegetable oil for greasing

CHEESECAKE

5 ounces white chocolate

10 ounces cream cheese, at room temperature

1 teaspoon pure vanilla extract or 1 vanilla bean

1 cup heavy cream

TOPPING

14 ounces mixed summer berries, such as strawberries, blackberries, raspberries, blueberries, and red currants

2 tablespoons seedless raspberry jam

2 ounces white chocolate

To make the crust, put the graham crackers in a plastic bag and crush them with a rolling pin; then mix with the melted butter. Press them into the bottom of a lightly oiled 8-inch loose-bottomed tart pan or springform pan (this can be done with a potato masher). Place in the refrigerator to chill.

Melt the white chocolate in a heatproof bowl over a pan of simmering water. Remove the bowl from the pan and beat in the cream cheese. Add the vanilla to the cream or, if using a vanilla bean, split it lengthwise with a sharp knife and scrape the seeds into the cream.

Whip the cream until it forms fairly stiff peaks and gently fold in the cream cheese and white chocolate mixture. Pour on top of the crust and put in the refrigerator for at least 2 hours to set.

Once the cake is set, carefully remove from the pan. Arrange the berries on top of the cake. Heat the jam with 2 teaspoons of water and strain through a sieve. Allow to cool for about 1 minute and gently brush over the fruits. Melt the white chocolate and drizzle over the top of the fruits with a teaspoon.

Summer berries *are packed with vitamin C, which helps to strengthen the immune system and fight infection. Vitamin C also aids in the absorption of iron.*

SUPERFOODS

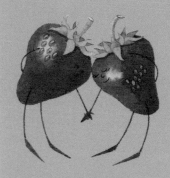

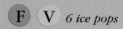
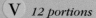
Strawberry sorbet ice pops

You can make delicious ice pops from fresh fruit.

$\frac{1}{3}$ **cup superfine sugar**
6 large strawberries, hulled and cut in half
Juice of 1 medium orange

Put the sugar and ¼ cup water into a saucepan; boil until syrupy (about 3 minutes). Let cool. Puree the strawberries and strain. Combine the strawberry puree, syrup, and orange juice and pour this mixture into ice pop molds. Freeze until solid.

Dark and white chocolate refrigerator cake

A tasty treat for children to make themselves.

7 ounces semisweet chocolate
$\frac{1}{3}$ **cup light corn syrup or golden syrup**
6 tablespoons unsalted butter
6 ounces graham crackers
$\frac{1}{2}$ **cup chopped dried apricots (about 12)**

$\frac{1}{4}$ **cup raisins**
$\frac{1}{2}$ **cup finely chopped pecans**
$1\frac{1}{2}$ **cups Rice Krispies**
3 ounces white chocolate, chopped into small pieces

Line a 9-inch square pan with plastic wrap, leaving enough to hang over the sides of the pan; this will help you remove the cake from the pan. Melt the semisweet chocolate, syrup, and butter in a heatproof bowl set over a pan of simmering water, making sure the bottom of the bowl does not touch the water. Stir occasionally until melted, then set aside to cool.

Break the graham crackers into small pieces, and mix together with the apricots, raisins, pecans, Rice Krispies, and white chocolate. Stir into the melted chocolate mixture. Spoon the mixture into the prepared pan and level the surface by pressing down gently with a potato masher or the back of a spoon. Place in the refrigerator until set, 1 to 2 hours. To serve, carefully peel off the plastic wrap and cut into 12 portions.

Cranberry, lemonade, and orange juice ice pops

F V *4 ice pops*

1 cup cranberry juice

½ cup lemonade

½ cup orange juice

Mix together all the ingredients. Pour into ice pop molds and freeze.

Cranberries *are rich in vitamin C—indeed, there is as much vitamin C in a glass of cranberry juice as in a glass of orange juice.*

My favorite carrot cake

F V *8 portions*

Can you think of a tastier way to eat your vegetables? And it's very easy to make.

1 cup vegetable oil, plus extra for greasing

1½ cups self-rising flour

¼ teaspoon baking powder

¼ teaspoon baking soda

Salt

1 teaspoon ground cinnamon

½ teaspoon ground ginger

2 large eggs, separated

2 cups light brown sugar, packed

1 cup grated carrot, packed
   (about 3 medium carrots)

½ cup crushed pineapple, drained

½ cup raisins

MAPLE CREAM CHEESE FROSTING

8 ounces cream cheese,
   at room temperature

1 stick unsalted butter, softened

½ cup confectioner's sugar

1 tablespoon maple syrup

Carrots *are rich in antioxidants, which are effective in supporting the body's immune system. One medium carrot will supply a six-year-old child's daily requirement of vitamin A.*

Preheat the oven to 325°F. Line and grease a 9-inch springform pan. Sift together the flour, baking powder, baking soda, a generous pinch of salt, the cinnamon, and ginger.

Whisk together the egg yolks, vegetable oil, and sugar. Whisk the egg whites with a pinch of salt until they stand in fairly firm peaks; set aside. Combine the egg yolk mixture with the dry ingredients. Stir in the carrot, pineapple, and raisins, then gently fold in half the egg whites and then the other half. (Don't feel you have to mix the egg whites in completely.)

Pour the mixture into the prepared pan and bake for 1 hour or until a skewer comes out clean when inserted in the center. Allow the cake to cool completely, then remove from the pan.

To make the frosting, beat the cream cheese with an electric mixer until light and smooth. In another bowl, beat the butter, sugar, and maple syrup together until light and fluffy. Fold this into the cream cheese. Spread the frosting on top of the cake and around the sides.

Cranberry juice *has long been used to help prevent and treat cystitis, and other bladder, kidney, and urinary tract infections. Cranberries are also a good source of vitamin C.*

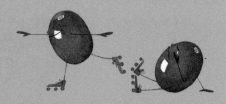

Tip: *Leaf gelatin is amazing—it dissolves like a dream every time, unlike powdered gelatin, which so often leaves stubborn little grains behind. You should be able to buy leaf gelatin in most large supermarkets or online.*

Cranberry-raspberry gelatin with summer fruits

This is a fantastic-looking dessert made with fresh fruit and fresh juice and it's very easy to prepare. You can either make one large gelatin or individual gelatins. If you can't find leaf gelatin, you could use one 1-ounce envelope of powdered gelatin.

6 leaves gelatin

2 cups cranberry-raspberry juice

1 cup superfine sugar

12 ounces mixed berries, such as blackberries, raspberries, blueberries, red currants, and strawberries (when fresh berries are out of season, you can use frozen berries)

RASPBERRY COULIS

1 cup raspberries

2 tablespoons confectioners' sugar, plus extra as needed

To make the gelatin, place the leaf gelatin or powdered gelatin (see headnote) in a shallow dish and pour in just enough cranberry-raspberry juice to cover the surface. Allow to soften for about 5 minutes.

Heat the remaining cranberry-raspberry juice and the sugar in a saucepan until piping hot. Mix in the softened gelatin and any juice, stirring until completely dissolved. Set aside to cool.

If using fresh fruit, halve the strawberries and remove the red currants from their stems. Rinse a 4-cup mold but do not dry (a wet mold will make it easier to remove the gelatin when it is set). You could also pour the gelatin into a loaf pan. Alternatively, divide the berries among 4 to 6 individual molds (or use glass dishes) and pour in the gelatin. Spoon in the fruit, pour in 1¼ cups of the gelatin, and leave in the refrigerator for about 1 hour or until beginning to set. When set, pour in the remaining gelatin to cover and return to the refrigerator to set.

To make the coulis, blitz the raspberries and sugar in a blender and push through a sieve to make a smooth sauce. Stir in extra sugar if necessary.

To turn out the gelatin, dip the mold into a bowl of hot water and run a knife around the edge of the mold or loaf pan to loosen the gelatin. Invert onto a large plate and give it a quick shake—the gelatin should slide out.

Serve the gelatin with a little raspberry coulis and maybe some vanilla ice cream.

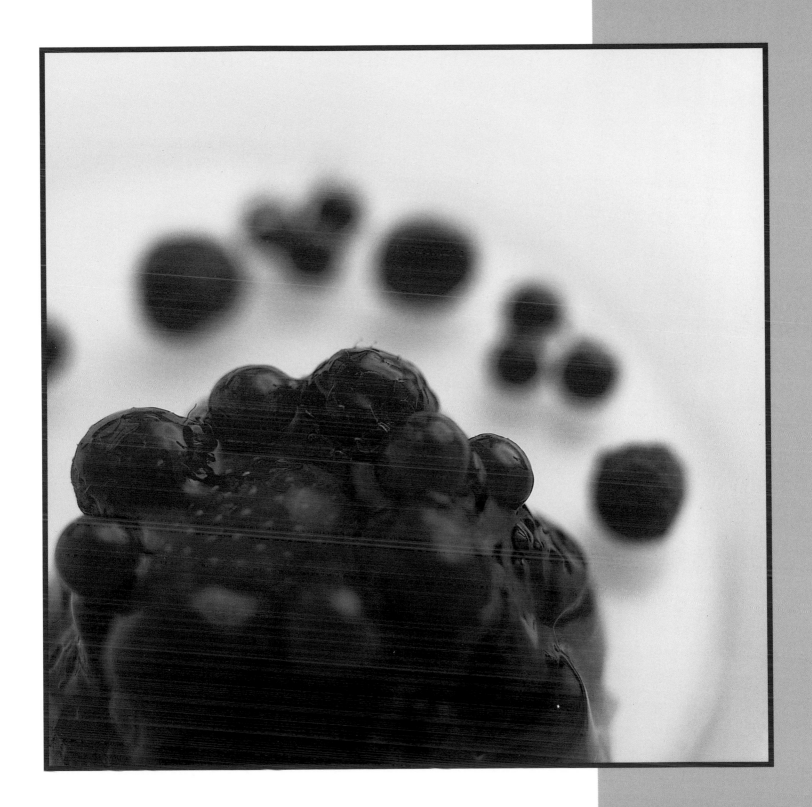

Oats *are high in soluble fiber, which helps lower blood cholesterol and also provides lasting energy, keeping hunger pangs at bay. Oatmeal is an ideal start to the day and should keep you full of energy.*

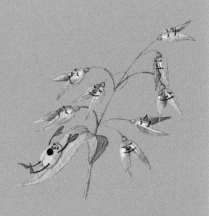

Apple, oat, and raisin muffins

These are known in my house as my one-legged muffins, as I made them after returning from a skiing vacation when I broke my leg. Luckily my two daughters, Lara and Scarlett, were very willing helpers in the kitchen, gathering together ingredients and helping me experiment until we collectively came up with this very delicious muffin recipe, which is now a family favorite.

1 egg
½ cup sunflower or canola oil
¾ cup whole milk
¾ cup rolled oats
1 cup all-purpose flour
3 teaspoons baking powder
½ cup superfine sugar
½ teaspoon salt
1 teaspoon pumpkin pie spice
½ teaspoon ground cinnamon
¾ cup raisins
1 apple, peeled, cored, and diced

Preheat the oven to 350°F. Beat the egg in a bowl and mix together with the oil and milk. In a large mixing bowl, mix together all the remaining ingredients. Pour in the egg mixture and mix until just moistened, taking care not to overmix. Pour into ten muffin cups lined with cupcake liners and bake for 25 minutes or until well risen and lightly golden.

Summer fruit yogurt ice cream

This creamy frozen yogurt tastes wonderful and is made with good healthy ingredients. You could also make it using fresh berries.

One 10-ounce package mixed frozen berries, such as raspberries, blackberries, blueberries, strawberries, cherries, and red currants, thawed (or use 2 cups fresh berries)
1¾ cups plain yogurt
1 cup heavy cream
¾ cup plus 1 tablespoon superfine sugar

Puree and strain half the berries. Stir the yogurt and lightly whisk the cream until it forms soft peaks. Mix together the yogurt, the cream, the ¾ cup sugar, and the berry puree. Freeze in an ice cream machine. When frozen, mix the remaining berries with the 1 tablespoon sugar and stir into the ice cream mixture.

Alternatively, spoon the yogurt mixture into a suitable container and put in the freezer. When half frozen, beat well until smooth, either with a handheld electric blender or in a food processor, to break down the ice crystals that form. Mix the rest of the berries with the 1 tablespoon sugar and stir into the yogurt ice cream. Return to the freezer and stir one or two more times during the freezing process to get a smooth ice cream.

Yogurt *can be used in place of milk if your child is lactose intolerant because the live bacteria used in the process of making yogurt have predigested a lot of the lactose (milk sugar) that causes problems in many people.*

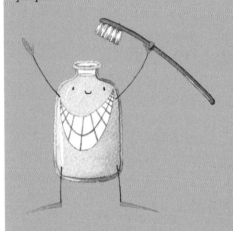

Summer fruit milkshake

One 12-ounce package mixed frozen berries, such as strawberries, blueberries, blackberries, cherries, and red currants, thawed (or use 2½ cups fresh berries)
½ cup confectioners' sugar
½ cup light cream
1 cup whole milk
Ice cubes

Puree and strain the berries and mix with the sugar. Stir in the light cream and milk. Serve in glasses over some ice cubes.

Milk *is great for children, as it is rich in calcium. Children will often drink milk when it is mixed with other foods, particularly fruit.*

Food allergies

Surveys show that as many as two in ten people believe they react badly to certain foods. However, a detailed British government study suggests that only about two in every one hundred people do have unpleasant reactions to food that can be measured. Many people blame food additives, but reactions to food additives are probably at least one hundred times less common than reactions to natural foods such as milk and wheat.

Food allergy generally begins in childhood and can trigger a wide range of symptoms from vomiting, persistent diarrhea, and abdominal pain to eczema, skin rashes, and wheezing. With so many symptoms that could have other causes, it is often hard to be sure that food is to blame or to find out which food. Reactions may occur immediately after eating a specific food or may be delayed for hours or even days. If you are worried that your child might be allergic to a certain food, you should seek expert medical advice.

An allergic reaction generally occurs when the immune system wrongly perceives a harmless substance as a threat and an immune response is triggered, producing a large amount of antibodies in the blood. This can cause or contribute to various conditions such as eczema, hives, hay fever, asthma, diarrhea, and even failure to thrive. With the later introduction of solid foods between four and six months, the incidence of food allergy in young babies has become less common. However, it is still babies under the age of eighteen months who are most likely to develop an allergy.

> **Healthy eating:** *Milk-free vegetable or soy margarine may be substituted for butter; there are also many soy-based (nondairy) yogurts and desserts available, and carob can be substituted for milk chocolate.*

The commonest foods that carry a risk of allergic reaction in babies

- Cow's milk and dairy products.
- Nuts.
- Eggs.
- Wheat-based products.
- Fish and shellfish.
- Citrus fruits and berries.

A family history of allergies

There is a lot of anxiety about food allergies. However, unless there is a family history of allergy, food allergies are quite rare. The risk of a child developing an allergic disorder more than doubles if there is a family history of a parent or sibling with an atopic disease such as asthma, eczema, or hay fever. In this case, breast-feeding for at least four, and preferably six, months seems to offer some protection. Bear in mind if you are breast-feeding that by eating certain foods like dairy products, eggs, oranges, and wheat, the allergic substances may be transmitted through your breast milk. This can then cause a reaction in your baby (like eczema). Don't cut out major food groups such as dairy products in your own diet, as you may become deficient yourself. Always check with a dietitian first.

Do not introduce any foods that might cause an allergy before six months at the earliest. Instead, start weaning with only low-allergen foods like baby rice, root vegetables, apple, and pear. Avoid high-risk foods (see list above) until your baby is nine to twelve months old. If there is a family history of allergy to a particular food, avoid that food until your child is at least one year old. Do not remove key foods from your child's diet without first consulting a doctor. If you suspect that your child is allergic to a common food such as milk or wheat, seek expert advice on planning a balanced diet.

Many children outgrow food allergies by three to five years. However, there is no cure for some lifelong allergies and the only way to remain healthy is to avoid the problem food. A young baby's immune system is not fully mature and babies can become ill very quickly, so never hesitate to call a doctor if you are worried.

How to diagnose a food allergy

The only accurate way to diagnose food allergies is to eliminate the suspected or most common allergens, wait for symptoms to cease, and after a period of about six weeks, reintroduce the foods one by one until the symptoms reappear. This is called an elimination diet followed by food challenging. This type of diet should be done only under medical supervision and with the help of a registered dietitian (RD). Other methods such as electrode testing and skin prick tests are not accurate means of diagnosing food allergies.

Specific food allergies

Cow's milk protein allergy: This is the most commonly occurring allergy in children. An allergic reaction to infant formula or any dairy product can occur in a matter of minutes, or even after a few days or weeks. Symptoms can include cramps, diarrhea, vomiting, a skin rash, or breathing difficulties.

If your baby is sensitive to cow's milk–based infant formula, consult your doctor, who might recommend either a soy-based formula or a specially designed hypoallergenic formula. About 30 percent of babies who are allergic to cow's milk also become allergic to soy milk. Breast milk is the best milk for babies, but breast-feeding mothers will need to eliminate dairy foods from their own diets.

If your child is allergic to cow's milk, make sure that any foods you buy do not contain: milk, butter, cheese, cream, yogurt, ghee, whey, lactose, or milk solids.

Food additives and colorings: Some widely used food additives, such as the food coloring Yellow No. 5, have been associated with allergic reactions in a small minority of children. There have also been reported links between hyperactivity and diet. There is some evidence that in a small minority (a much lower incidence than is perceived by parents), additives such as flavorings and coloring or foods such as milk and wheat may change behavior.

Food intolerance: A food intolerance, sometimes called a false food allergy, is a condition where the body is temporarily incapable of digesting certain foods. It is generally short-lived and is not the same as a true food allergy, which involves the immune system. However, it can provoke the same symptoms, so if you suspect that your child is allergic to a common food like cow's milk, you should consult your pediatrician before changing milk formula. It is quite possible that your baby's reaction is only temporary. If your child is found to be allergic to a basic food like wheat, you should always seek expert advice as to how you can keep meals balanced.

Gluten intolerance: Gluten is found in wheat, rye, barley, and oats and is therefore present in foods like bread, pasta, and cookies. Some people suffer from a permanent sensitivity to gluten—a condition known as celiac disease—which, although rare, is a serious medical condition. It is diagnosed medically by a blood test and confirmed by actually looking at the gut wall using endoscopy.

Symptoms of celiac disease include loss of appetite, poor growth, swollen abdomen, and pale, bulky, frothy, and smelly stools. Foods containing gluten should not be introduced into any baby's diet before six months. Cereals used between four and six months should be gluten free, such as rice and corn. When buying baby cereals and zwiebacks, choose varieties that are gluten free. Baby rice is the safest to try at first, and thereafter there are plenty of alternative gluten-free products such as soy, corn, rice, millet, rice noodles, buckwheat spaghetti, and potato flours for thickening and baking.

Peanuts: Peanuts and peanut products can induce a severe allergic reaction called anaphylactic shock, which can be life threatening. In families with a history of any allergy, including hay fever, eczema, and asthma, it is advisable to avoid all products containing peanuts until the child is three years old and then seek medical advice before introducing peanut products into the diet. Vegetable oils, which may contain peanut oil, will not cause a reaction, as the oil is refined, removing any traces of peanut protein. Provided there is no family history of allergy, peanut butter and finely ground nuts can be introduced from six months. Whole nuts should not be given to children under the age of five because of the risk of choking.

Foods for common ailments

Asthma
See Atopic illnesses.

Atopic illnesses
Breast-feeding will help delay the onset of any of the atopic-type illnesses such as asthma, eczema, food allergies, and hay fever. In some cases, dietary changes may alleviate the symptoms, but the only way to be certain is to follow an elimination diet.

Colds and flu
Make sure your child has plenty of fresh fruit and vegetables to ensure a good intake of vitamins and minerals. Look especially to those rich in vitamin C (see page 16). Recent research shows that chicken soup can help reduce mucus, boost immunity, and reduce inflammation in the nose—it is easy to swallow and rich in vitamins and minerals.

Colic
Colic is common in babies between six weeks and three months and often is worse in the evenings. The causes of colic are still uncertain, but to help alleviate symptoms, some breast-feeding mothers eliminate certain foods from their diets. If individual foods such as raspberries are eliminated, this is fine, but if major food groups such as dairy products are eliminated, dietetic advice should be sought immediately. Eliminating dairy products, a major source of calcium during breast-feeding, puts a mother at risk of developing serious problems such as osteoporosis, or weak bones, when she is older.

Coping with colic
• Changing the feeding position of your baby to a more upright position and gentle movement may help to settle some babies.
• Alcohol-free gripe water preparations may be given over one month of age.
• Colic drops may be useful.

• Herbal drinks may be given in small amounts as long as they are sugar free (remember, "dextrose" means "sugar").
• Massage can help to relieve pain and tension.

Constipation
Constipation is the infrequent passing of hard stools every four to eight days. It is very rare in breast-fed infants, as breast milk is more easily digested and has a laxative effect. Formula-fed infants tend to pass stools less frequently and the stools can be a different color and consistency. Babies' bowel habits vary, but if you think your baby is constipated, first try ensuring feedings are made up properly and not overconcentrated and offer bottles of cooled boiled water between milk feedings. Do not add sugar to the feeding bottle, as this could make things worse.

Once your baby is weaned, give foods that are naturally rich in fiber, such as fruit and vegetables, prunes (fruit and juice), and baked beans and lentils. After she is six months old, avoid giving refined foods like white bread and sugary breakfast cereals and give whole-grain bread and whole-grain cereals like oatmeal and muesli instead. Offer chopped nuts and dried fruit and use whole-wheat pasta and brown rice. Avoid binding food like rice pudding and macaroni and cheese. If the problem persists and is severe, see your pediatrician.

Diarrhea
Most children suffer with diarrhea at some point; it is a sign that the body needs to evacuate something that is causing irritation, and it may be accompanied by vomiting. There are many possible reasons for diarrhea. It may be caused by too much fiber or fruit juice in the diet, or it may indicate a food sensitivity or some kind of food poisoning. Diarrhea can also be a side effect of drugs, particularly antibiotics.

Most children will lose their appetites to some degree when they are unwell. Young children can become seriously dehydrated very quickly, so the important thing is to make sure your child is maintaining his fluid intake. Continue to offer milk feedings and cooled boiled water. Very diluted fruit juice can also be used. For babies over six weeks add 1 teaspoon unsweetened fruit juice or baby fruit juice to 2 tablespoons cooled boiled water; for babies over three months add 2 to 3 teaspoons unsweetened fruit juice to 2 tablespoons cooled boiled water.

If the diarrhea persists, then you can try some oral rehydration fluid from your pharmacist to prevent dehydration. If your baby or child is vomiting as well and unable to keep anything down, then contact your pediatrician for further advice.

Sometimes when a child has had diarrhea for an extended period, he may develop a secondary lactose intolerance. This means that he may become intolerant to the sugar in the milk. This is usually a temporary condition and will resolve by itself once the diarrhea is improved. Do not stop milk feedings for infants without consulting a health professional first. Babies with diarrhea still need fluid and nutrition, and milk provides both.

Good foods to give your child once the diarrhea has stopped include rice, semolina, broiled fish, banana and toast, plain cookies, and apple puree (see recipe on page 40).

Eczema

Eczema is a complicated subject and children with eczema should always be checked out by their pediatrician. There is also an eczema Web site, which provides information and advice for sufferers and their families. Eczema is often due not to food but to other things, such as laundry detergents, soaps, grasses, or pollens in the air. If a child has an allergic family, then breast-feeding may help delay the onset of eczema. The foods most commonly implicated in food allergies that may present as eczema are cow's milk, nuts, wheat, eggs, and shellfish (see also pages 184 to 185).

Fever

When your child is unwell and off her food, always give plenty of fluids. Try offering nourishing fluids like milk-based drinks such as hot chocolate and milkshakes. Clear soups, especially chicken soup, are also good.

Offer your child her favorite foods to stimulate her appetite, but don't get too worried. Minimal food for a few days will not have a serious impact on your child's health and most children will make up for it by eating more than usual when they are better.

If your child is on antibiotics, offer live yogurt. Antibiotics kill off both bad and good bacteria in the intestine and eating live yogurt helps restore the good bacteria.

Food allergies

See Atopic illnesses and pages 184 to 185.

Gas

See Colic.

Hay fever

See Atopic illnesses.

Lactose intolerance

Lactose intolerance is sometimes—incorrectly—thought to be an allergy. In fact, lactose is the sugar in milk and lactose intolerance is the inability to digest this sugar because of a lack of a digestive enzyme called lactase in the gut. The main symptoms are diarrhea, cramping, flatulence, and abdominal distension. Lactose intolerance can be hereditary, in which the body simply does not produce a sufficient amount of lactase, or lactose intolerance can follow a period of gastroenteritis (infection in the gut). Following gastroenteritis, the sites where the enzyme lactase is produced may be damaged and therefore the lactose remains undigested, causing problems. In a few weeks to months, the enzyme begins to be produced again and lactose is digested normally again.

Children with lactose intolerance should avoid dairy products and either consume at least 20 ounces of calcium-fortified soy milk daily plus calcium-rich foods or take a calcium supplement, which can be prescribed by their doctor. Recently low-lactose formulas and low-lactose milks have been designed for lactose intolerance.

Index

A

additives, food, 22, 185

allergies, food, 28, 30, 184–85, 186, 187

antioxidants, 10, 13, 16, 22

apples, 70; Apple, Oat, and Raisin Muffins, 182; purees, 38, 40, 42, 46, 64, 65

apricots, 12, 20, 45

apricots, dried, 20, 45, 46, 70; My Favorite Oatmeal, 65; purees, 46, 64

asthma, 184, 186

attention deficit disorder, 17

avocados, 77; Creamy Avocado Dip, 77; purees, 40, 42

B

bananas, 19, 42, 64, 70; purees, 40, 42, 64

basil, 171

beef, 166; Beef in Hoisin Sauce with Broccoli and Water Chestnuts, 129; Braised Beef with Carrot, Parsnip, and Sweet Potato, 44; Meatballs with Sweet-and Sour Sauce, 102; Mild Beef Curry, 167; Mini Shepherd's Pie, 83; My Favorite Beefburgers, 166; Old-fashioned Beef Casserole, 60; spaghetti Bolognese, 85, 104; Stir-fried Shredded Beef, 166

beets, 12

beta-carotene, 10, 12

blackberries, 111, *see also* summer fruits

blueberries, 12, 13, 46, *see also* summer fruits; puree, 46

bread, 13, 19, 86, 91, 133; Cheat's Cheese Soufflé, 133; French Toast, 86

breakfasts (1–2 yrs), 90–91

breast-feeding, 28, 185

broccoli, 29, 43, 74, 75, 129; Broccoli in Cheese Sauce, 75; Chicken and Broccoli Salad, 124; purees, 43, 57

brownies, 142

burgers, 115, 128, 166, 170, 172

butternut squash, 29, 38, 44; Cheesy Baked Potato with Butternut Squash, 132; Fruity Chicken with Butternut Squash, 59; purees, 38, 44; Risotto with Butternut Squash, 81

C

cabbage, 119

calcium, 14, 16, 20, 69, 90

canned food, 23

carbohydrates, 13, 17, 19, 22

carotenoids, 12, 14

carrots, 12, 29, 36, 44, 74, 96, 179; Carrot, Cheese, and Tomato Risotto, 74; Carrot Soup with Yellow Split Peas, 96; Mashed Potato and Carrot with Broccoli and Swiss Cheese, 74; My Favorite Carrot Cake, 179; purees, 36, 38, 39, 45, 54, 61, 62

cauliflower, 29, 43, 62; purees, 62

cereals, 13, 16, 17, 30, 50, 68, 91, 185

cheese, 14, 16, 17, 30, 50, 69, 72, 81, 94, 127; Broccoli in Cheese Sauce, 75; Carrot, Cheese, and Tomato Risotto, 74; Cheat's Cheese Soufflé, 133; Cheese and Zucchini Sausages, 100; Cheesy Baked Potato with Butternut Squash, 132; Cheesy Mushroom and Tomato Sauce with Pasta Stars, 75; Cream Cheese, Tomato, and Chive Dip, 77; Crispy Cheese, Cabbage, and Potato Bake, 119; Mashed Potato and Carrot with Broccoli and Swiss Cheese, 74; Mixed Berry and White Chocolate Cheesecake, 177; Rabbit Muffins, 94; Spinach and Ricotta Cannelloni, 127; Spinach, Cheese, and Tomato Lasagne, 171; Tiny Pasta with Swiss Cheese, Spinach, and Corn, 72; Vegetable Puree with Tomato and Cheese, 62

Cherry and Banana Puree, 64

Cherub's Couscous, 78

chicken, 59, 100, 101, 128, 164; Annabel's Chicken Dippers, 122; Annabel's Tasty Chicken Skewers, 101; Chicken and Broccoli Salad, 124; Chicken Cannelloni, 162; Chicken Fingers Marinated in Buttermilk, 156; Chicken Noodle Soup, 154; Chicken Salad with Corn, Pasta, and Cherry Tomatoes, 118; Chicken with Matchsticks, 100; Chopped Chicken with Diced Vegetables in Cheese

M

mangoes, 12; Tropical Treat, 143

mascarpone, 122

meat, 14, 16, 17, 29, 50, 51, 83, 85, 92, 102, 104, *see also* beef; chicken; lamb; veal

Meatballs with Sweet-and-Sour Sauce, 102

melons, 12, 45

milk, 14, 16, 50, 68, 80, 92, 185, 187; breast, 17, 28, 50, 68; formula 28, 50, 68; soy, 20; Summer Fruit Milkshake, 183

minerals, 14, 16, *see also* iron

muffins, 94, 182

N

Nasi Goreng, 155

nectarines, 45; smoothie, 143

noodles, stir-fried, 122, 130

nuts, 16, 19, 20, 30, 52, 170, 184, 185, *see also* peanuts

O

oats, 65, 185; Apple, Oat, and Raisin Muffins, 182; Apple, Pear, and Prune with Oats, 65; Chewy Oatmeal Raisin Cookies, 146; oatmeal, 17, 19, 65

obesity, 115–16

oils, 17, 19, 185; olive, 120, 156

onions, 13, 132, 172

organic foods, 24

organosulphides, 13

orzo: Orzo Risotto, 96; Orzo with Creamy Mushroom and Cheese Sauce, 81

P

papayas, 12, 40; purees, 40, 64

parsnips, 29, 38, 44; Oven-Fried Root Vegetables, 107; purees, 36, 38, 54

pasta, 13, 16, 19, 80, 96; Bow-tie Pasta with Salmon and Tomatoes, 139; Bow-tie Pasta Salad with Tuna, 134; cannelloni, 127, 162; Pasta Risotto, 80; spaghetti Bolognese, 85, 104; Spinach, Cheese, and Tomato Lasagne, 171; Tiny Pasta with Spinach, Corn, and Swiss Cheese, 72; Tuna Tagliatelle, 138

peaches, 12, 20, 45, 64, 70; Fresh Peach Melba, 85; ice pops, 108, 146; Mixed Berry and Peach Crumble, 174; Peach Melba Frozen Yogurt with Crushed Meringues, 145; smoothies, 111, 143

peanut butter, 90, 157, 159

peanuts, 185

pears, 42; purees, 40, 42, 44, 46, 65

peas, 29, 57; purees, 57, 61

pectin, 40

peppers, bell, 12, 16, 52, 118; Special Tomato Pasta Sauce, 118

Pilau Rice, 161

plums, 45

potatoes, 12, 13, 16, 19, 61, 134; Cheesy Baked Potato with Butternut Squash, 132; Crispy Cheese, Cabbage, and Potato Bake, 119; Mashed Potato and Carrot with Broccoli and Swiss Cheese, 74; Oven-Fried Root Vegetables, 107; purees, 36, 45; rösti, 163; Spinach with Mushrooms and Potato, 72; Vegetable Croquettes, 134

potatoes, sweet, 12, 17, 29, 39, 44, 54, 107; Oven-Fried Root Vegetables, 107; purees, 36, 39, 43, 54

protein, 14, 17, 20

prunes, 65

purees, making, 30–31

R

Rabbit Muffins, 94

raisins, 146

raspberries, 30, 77, 85, 108, *see also* summer fruits; Fresh Peach Melba, 85; Peach Melba Smoothie, 111; Peach Melba Frozen Yogurt with Crushed Meringues, 145; Peach, Strawberry, and Raspberry Ice Pops, 108; Raspberry Yogurt Dip, 77

rejection, food, 30

rice, 13, 17, 19, 106, 123; baby, 29, 39, 42, 44; Brown Rice with Diced Vegetables, 97; Chinese Fried Rice, 123; Pilau Rice, 161; Rice 'n' Easy, 106; Risotto with Butternut Squash, 81; Strawberry Rice Pudding, 86

rösti, 163

rutabagas, 29, 36

Acknowledgments

To my three children, Nicholas, Lara, and Scarlett, who have chomped through the pages of this book with gusto.

To my husband, Simon, whose expertise in the eating of baby food is unsurpassed.

To my mother, Evelyn Etkind, who frequently raids my fridge for the benefit of her dinner parties.

To David Karmel for his late-night rescue missions to retrieve my day's output from the recycle bin.

To Daniel Pangbourne for his fabulous photography. He brings food to life and manages to keep children still.

To Jacqui Barnett for her tireless support and enthusiasm.

To Judith Curr, Greer Hendricks, Kim Yorio, Sybil Pincus, Virginia McRae, Annette Corkey, and Hannah Morrill at Atria Books.

To Marina Magpoc, Letty Catada, and Jane Hamilton, a special big thank you for all your help.

To Gail Rebuck, Emma Callery, Helen Lewis, Sarah Lewis, Tessa Evelegh, Jo Pratt, Borra Garson, and Stephen Springate.

To my wonderful models, Amelia Arkhurst, Louis Fattal, Somerset Francis, Jo Glick, Scarlett Karmel, Lucas Keusey, Olivia Leigh, Anouska Levy, Alexandra Meller, Harry Ross, and Arabella Schild.

The publishers would also like to thank the following for the loan of props in this book: Heal's, 196 Tottenham Court Road, London W1P 9LD and branches (nursery furniture); Muji, 6 Tottenham Court Road, London W1 and branches (baby clothes), Babygap, branches countrywide (baby clothes) and Bridgewater, 739 Fulham Road, London SW6 5UL (pottery).

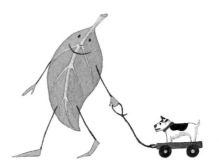

Annabel Karmel is the mother of three children, a bestselling author of more than twenty books on nutrition and cooking for babies and toddlers, and the UK's leading expert on feeding children. She is the food writer for *Scholastic Parent & Child* magazine, and works with leading U.S. parenting websites including Family.com, Sesame Street, and Baby Center. Annabel has also appeared on many TV programs, including the *Today* show, *The Early Show,* and *The View.* Please visit her website at www.annabelkarmel.com.